THE
BREASTFEEDING SOURCEBOOK

OTHER BOOKS BY M. SARA ROSENTHAL

The Thyroid Sourcebook, 3d edition

The Gynecological Sourcebook, 2d edition

The Pregnancy Sourcebook, 2d edition

The Fertility Sourcebook, 2d edition

The Breast Sourcebook

The Gastrointestinal Sourcebook

THE
BREASTFEEDING
SOURCEBOOK

Everything You Need to Know

Second Edition

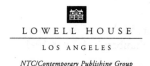

M. SARA ROSENTHAL

with a foreword by
Gillian Arsenault, M.D., M.H.Sc., I.B.C.L.C., F.R.C.P.

LOWELL HOUSE

LOS ANGELES

NTC/Contemporary Publishing Group

The purpose of this book is to educate. It is sold with the understanding that the author and Lowell House shall have neither liability nor responsibility for any injury caused or alleged to be caused directly or indirectly by the information contained in this book. While every effort has been made to ensure its accuracy, the book's contents should not be construed as medical advice. Each person's health needs are unique. To obtain recommendations appropriate to your particular situation, please consult a qualified health care provider.

LIBRARY OF CONGRESS CATALOGING-IN-PUBLICATION DATA

Rosenthal, M. Sara.
    The breastfeeding sourcebook : everything you need to know / by M. Sara Rosenthal : with a foreword by Gillian Arsenault.
        p.   cm.
    Includes bibliographical references and index.
    ISBN 1-56565-342-4 (hardcover)
    ISBN 1-56565-478-1 (paper)
    ISBN 0-7373-0019-1 (2d ed.)
    1. Breastfeeding.   I. Title.
    RJ216.R577   1995
    649'.33—dc20   95-31394
                                                                  CIP

Requests for such permissions should be addressed to:
Lowell House
2020 Avenue of the Stars, Suite 300
Los Angeles, CA 90067

Published by Lowell House,
a division of NTC/Contemporary Publishing Group, Inc.
4255 West Touhy Avenue, Lincolnwood, Illinois 60646-1975 U.S.A.

Design by Kate Mueller

Printed and bound in the United States of America
International Standard Book Number: 0-7373-0019-1

10 9 8 7 6 5 4 3 2 1

To Kayla and Jacob

CONTENTS

$\mathcal{A}$CKNOWLEDGMENTS

If it weren't for the commitment, hard work, and guidance of the following people, this book would never have been written: Gillian Arsenault, M.D., F.R.C.P., C.C.F.P., I.B.C.L.C., who served as medical adviser and provided me with so many valuable resources and materials; my research assistants, Ellen Tulchinsky, B.A., M.L.I.S., Laura Tulchinsky, B.A., Larissa Kostoff, and Sujata Talreja; my editor, Bud Sperry, and my copy editor, Kate Zentall.

Special thanks to the physicians and health practitioners who donated their time and expertise: Sue Johanson, R.N., sex educator and counselor; Masood A. Khatamee, M.D., F.A.C.O.G.; Debra Lander, M.D., F.R.C.P. (C); Matthew Lazar, M.D., F.R.C.P. (C), F.A.C.P; Michelle Long, M.D.; Kelly S. MacDonald, M.D, F.R.C.P. (C); Frank Pratt, M.D., F.A.C.P, and especially Suzanne Pratt, M.D., F.A.C.O.G., who provided so much of the groundwork for this text.

I'd also like to thank La Leche League Canada and all of the mothers I interviewed. Your stories, struggles, and important suggestions regarding the content for this book were very much appreciated.

In the moral support department: my husband, Gary S. Karp, and all the relatives and friends who cheered me on.

$\mathcal{F}$OREWORD

Welcome to the wonderful world of parenthood! For some, this will be the first venture into a new, rich, and challenging land; for others, it is well-loved and familiar territory. The book you hold in your hands is a treasure map. The treasure dealt with here is breastfeeding, and all the medial, psychological—and yes—economical benefits that come with it.

Lest you think I exaggerate, this is what UNICEF has to say about breastfeeding:

"Imagine that the world had invented a new 'dream product' to feed and immunize everyone on Earth. Imagine also that it was available everywhere, required no storage or delivery, and helped mothers to plan their families and reduce the risk of cancer. Then imagine that the world refused to use it. The 'dream product' is human breastmilk, available to us all at birth, and yet we are not using it."

Our culture has, in general, forgotten how to breastfeed. Breastfeeding is a learned skill, not an instinct. Our mothers and infants must learn anew to travel the breastfeeding path, and many are the pitfalls that our technological, consumerist society places in the way of the innocent and unwary. In this, as in all journeys, the knowledge and wisdom of those who have gone before us can make the trip much easier.

M. Sara Rosenthal, the author of this book, has done what many of us do when we first become pregnant. She has sought out and talked to numerous mothers, and read what they have written; and she has consulted physicians and the scientific literature. The results you hold in your hand: a compilation of valuable information, a guide, a map.

Your own individual journey as a mother will be unique and your very own. Some of you will be blessed with a journey of breathless ease, through a safe haven free of formula samples and artificial nipples. You will have a baby that takes to your breast from birth. You will have friends and family who know how the rest of the world breastfeeds and applaud and support the priceless gift you give your child. For you, reading this book is like getting travel insurance; you wouldn't journey without it, but you're delighted to discover that you didn't really need it.

Some of you, through absolutely no fault of your own, will face stormy weather and wolves howling in the woods. You will need the information in this book, and perhaps more besides. The author has included suggestions for finding further information and assistance, that may be required. For those of you who do face the storms, as I did myself with my first child, I would like to offer one small word of comfort: it gets easier! When the thrush is treated and the latch corrected, when the causes of low milk supply are removed, the mastitis cleared, the anemia resolved—ah, it becomes so much easier to find the joy you had been expecting. And the longer you breastfeed, the easier it gets, and the closer and the more immediate is the joy. The only challenge is then coming up with snappy comebacks to deal with the well-intentioned but ill-informed who think that the journey of breastfeeding should end far too early.

And for those of you who face storms that cannot be endured, heights that cannot be scaled, please remember that all of us (even mothers) are only human. We can only do what we can do. Your love for your child that led you to undertake the journey, and your courage that sustained you in the struggles are also treasures, priceless gifts that you give to your child. You may read this book, only to discover that you could not continue because you were given no information, or worse, the wrong information, or because there was no support to be had. If this has happened to you, you may well look askance at those who should have been there to help. All too often, physicians are able to fix hearts but not sore nipples. And our society is willing to accommodate people in wheelchairs, but not nursing mothers. None of this is your fault.

I am one of those physicians who knew nothing about breastfeeding because it was not taught when I went to medical school. Then I had a baby, and I learned. I learned from my child, and I learned from other mothers who had breastfed. Eventually, I realized that there was a vast body of scientific information about breastfeeding that my medical school had been steadfastly ignoring. So I went to the medical literature and learned about the breastfeeding research, too.

And the interesting thing was, that the science only confirmed what I had been taught by other breastfeeding mothers, and by my own children.

I wish you all a joyful journey into parenting, and into breastfeeding. May your path be always smooth, and may the wind be ever at your back!

GILLIAN ARSENAULT,
M.D., M.H.Sc., I.B.C.L.C., F.R.C.P.

I HOPE YOU HAVEN'T DELIVERED YET

If breastfeeding is so normal and natural, why do we need to be taught how to breastfeed? Why doesn't it come naturally to every woman? Well, childbirth is natural, too. But without any instruction or guidance, would you know instinctively how to deliver a baby? Would you be able to deliver your own baby in the woods?

A hundred years ago, breastfeeding did come naturally to most women. Yet as urbanization grew, so did the bottle-feeding trend. You can probably track the decline of breastfeeding in this century by doing a maternal "family tree," which may look something like this:

1896: Great-grandmother was born and breastfed
1916: Grandmother was born and breastfed
1935: Aunt was born and breastfed
1939: Uncle was born and breastfed
1943: Mother was born and bottle-fed
1963: You were born and bottle-fed

Some crucial facts to remember about the above family tree is that the great-grandmother was maybe the tenth of thirteen children; the grandmother, the fourth of seven children; and the mother, as indicated, the youngest of three children. If you were born at the tail end of the baby boom, you probably have no more than three siblings—all of whom were bottle-fed too. It's a classic case of monkey see, monkey do. Your great-grandmother witnessed the art and technique of breastfeeding from her mother, who witnessed it from *her* mother, and so on. With large, double-digit families, your great-grandmother was able to witness the breastfeeding of three more siblings younger than herself. Even the youngest girl in this family saw the neighbors breastfeed, or her older sisters breastfeed her nieces and nephews. Your grandmother was also familiar with the technique, witnessing her younger siblings' feedings. As for your mother, she was born in a modern hospital, where your grandmother was taught how "modern mothers" fed their babies. So your mother, the youngest in her family, had no way of witnessing breastfeeding and learning the technique. By the time our own generation was born, hardly any of us was breastfed. (Worse, many of our mothers smoked during pregnancy, too.) As you can see, it took only one generation for breastfeeding to become a lost instinct.

Prior to 1900, 100 percent of all North American women breastfed their children, or had them breastfed by wet nurses. By 1950, roughly 60 percent of all North American women breastfed their first-born children; by 1960, only about 37 percent were breastfeeding; and by 1970, breastfeeding had declined even more, to just 27 percent of all first-time mothers breastfeeding. Finally, at an all-time low, only 7 percent of babies born between 1971 and 1973 were breastfed for three months or more.

Well, now it's the turn of the century again (not to mention the millennium), and we've learned that abandoning breastfeeding was a big mistake. The American Academy of Pediatrics (AAP) Work Group on Breastfeeding currently recommends breast milk as the preferred source of nutrition for almost all babies at least during the first year of life and for as long as mutually desired by mother and baby. The AAP's 1982 recommendation for breastfeeding was six to twelve months. (However, the new recommendations are still half of what the World Health Organization recommends to mothers.) The AAP also recommends that breastfeeding should occur within the first hour after birth; a trained observer should ensure that breastfeeding is going well during the first three days after birth (twenty-four to forty-eight hours after delivery and during a follow-up visit forty-eight to seventy-two hours after discharge); no plain or sugar water or formula be given to newborns unless medically indicated; and mothers provide expressed breast milk for their babies when nursing them directly is not possible. As a result, breastfeeding has dramatically risen in popularity. Much of this has to do with the abundance of medical literature supporting the nutritional benefits of breastfeeding for both baby and *you,* which we'll discuss further in chapter 2. This has led to a turnaround in breast-feeding counseling from the medical community, which advises doctors to tell their patients that breastfeeding is preferable to formula feeding and to plan for it, if possible. Some other reasons why breastfeeding is gaining popularity has to do with a larger societal shift away from manufactured products and toward all things natural. People are also waking up to the fact that baby humans are not baby cows, and therefore should be drinking human milk, rather than formula or cow's milk.

Unfortunately, even though most health care practitioners recognize the dangers of not breastfeeding, most of the information available to maternity and obstetrical patients about breastfeeding is actually wrong. Moreover, Dr. Gillian Arsenault, the medical adviser for this book, relates, as a doctor she wasn't taught anything at all about breastfeeding in medical school, and didn't realize how ignorant she was about breastfeeding until she herself had a child. Many published and accepted books on breastfeeding that are currently in bookstores acutally contain outdated material or misinformation. For example, "feeding schedules," "calories per baby," and "rubber nipple shields" are obsolete concerns and concepts offered in several current breastfeeding books that are antithetical to a good breastfeeding experience. The book you have in hand has been designed to work for a *real* woman with *real* breasts, who *really* wants to breastfeed. No assumptions are made about any previous knowledge you may have of breast functions and breastfeeding, since, like the rest of us, much of what you may have learned may be wrong. So chapter 1, entitled "Breasts 101," starts at the beginning. It explains exactly how the breasts develop and work, what the "lactation hormones" oxytocin and prolactin do, and the kinds of physiological oddities that can occur, such as inverted nipples. Chapter 1 also discusses the sexual purpose of the breast and the breast self-exam (BSE), something that all women over twenty should be practicing on a monthly basis. (Yes, you *can* develop breast cancer while you're lactating, just as you can at other times in your life.) It's crucial to understand how your breasts work if you're actually going to use them.

Chapter 2, "Making the Decision," is the chapter to read if you're undecided about breastfeeding or unsure about whether you should be breastfeeding. Remember, we're a cancer-ravaged society, with many first-time mothers who are cancer survivors and breast-implant wearers. Many women are taking medications on a daily basis that could pass into their breast milk; other women are HIV-positive, or fear that they may be; many women suffer from chronic diseases, such as diabetes, lupus, or rheumatoid arthritis. Some women are also unclear about the true benefits of breast-feeding, and what breastfeeding demands in terms of time, commitment, and diet. I'll uncover the breastfeeding myths and separate truth from fiction. I'll also open up the political can of worms surrounding the breast-feeding vs. bottle-feeding debate. In essence, chapter 2 will help you make the decision that's right for you, providing guidelines for who is—and who isn't—a breastfeeding candidate.

Chapter 3, "Preparing for Breastfeeding," will outline everything you can do to facilitate a good breastfeeding experience from the outset. This includes finding a lactation consultant, the right doctor or midwife prior to delivery to discuss breastfeeding, anticipating problems in advance, such as twin (or more) feedings or dealing with inverted nipples, looking into breast pumps in advance if you plan to go back to work, and making sure that your hospital is baby friendly. You'll also find out how to make arrangements on your birth plan (if you have one) to ensure a proper start.

Breastfeeding veterans will appreciate chapter 4, because it is the chapter they most wish they had had during *their* first week. The first week of breastfeeding is the most important; if you don't get the hang of feeding here, you may be tempted to give up. (And many women have, because they lacked some simple information.) That's why I've devoted an entire chapter to this crucial time. You'll find everything you need to know about getting started, latching on, overcoming problems, and so on. If nothing else, read *this*!

Chapter 5, "Expressing Yourself," contains key information about long-term breastfeeding management. Even if things don't go as well as planned during your first week, regular milk expression/pumping is the best way to keep up a milk supply. It's also important to understand when to express/pump milk and store it so that you can supplement feedings, should you need to. Chapter 5 also discusses issues surrounding relactation. This brings us to chapter 6, "When to Supplement," which also explores alternate feeding tools that will not interfere with breastfeeding.

Chapter 7, "When Nursing Hurts," discusses the cause of pain while breastfeeding, such as a bad latch, an engorged breast, or infection. Diagnosis and treatment for a variety of breast and nipple ailments are examined.

When your breastfed baby is fussy or ill, chapter 8, "Growing Pains: Common and Not-So-Common Infant Ailments" is the one to read. Everything from colic, jaundice, slow weight gain, and "nursing strike" is covered alphabetically (in the Baby-C's section), while separate sections on allergies, common infections, and hospitalization are provided.

Planning to go back to work? Then make sure you read chapter 9, "Breastfeeding in the Workplace." The workplace is not a very lactation-friendly environment. But here you'll find all kinds of practical tips on overcoming obstacles, including how to make deals with coworkers, where to find comfortable, private places to pump, how to bring existing legislation that supports breastfeeding in the workplace to the attention of your employer, and ways to lobby for a mother-friendly environment. Finally, if you fear that you're exposed to toxins at work that could affect your own health—and your breast milk—this chapter discusses the truly unsafe work environments that you'll need to avoid, unless you plan to stop breastfeeding.

Chapter 10, "Sex and the Breastfeeding Woman," is all about breastfeeding, sexuality, and fertility. How does breastfeeding affect your sex life, your contraceptive choices, and your menstrual cycle? And what about breastfeeding during pregnancy and tandem nursing (nursing two children of different ages)? You'll find out!

Chapter 11, "What You Should Know About Baby Milk," is crucial reading for every mother. It's important to understand why we think it's "normal" to feed something artificial to a baby, yet abnormal to breastfeed. This chapter explains how we arrived at that kind of thinking.

Finally, I've provided a list of lay organizations, milk banks, and peer support groups you can contact for help with breastfeeding preparation and consultation.

The information in this book is correct and completely current as of this writing. Much of what you'll find here has not been published before. Use it, read it, and share it with other lactating women. *Bon appetit!*

chapter 1

BREASTS 101

I f you're like most women, until your first pregnancy the focus of your attention was all below the belt. In your teens, you worried about preventing pregnancy. Once you decided to have a child, you concentrated on getting pregnant and learning all about your ovulation cycle. If you're pregnant as a result of fertility treatments, you're most likely an expert on your reproductive system. But until your final weeks of pregnancy, you probably never really thought about your breasts as anything more than cosmetic instruments of sexual attraction.

Breasts are an amazing piece of glandular equipment. You may be familiar with the term *endocrine gland*. Well, the breasts are called *exocrine glands* because they produce a product that is used *outside* of your bloodstream. In the case of breasts, the product they make is not one that your own body uses, but one that continues the work of the placenta, nourishing your baby.

The purpose of this chapter is to not only give you the inside story of the breast but to introduce some of the common anatomical obstacles women encounter when they enter the mysterious world of breastfeeding—a place most women never knew existed.

LET'S TAKE IT FROM THE TOP

You probably grew up with very little information about how your breasts develop and work, so let's take it, as they say, from the top.

Normally, when we think of our reproductive organs, we think of our pelvic contents—the uterus, fallopian tubes, and ovaries. But the breasts are an integral part of that reproductive system. The technical purpose for breasts is to produce milk to feed a baby, but anthropologists believe that they serve an important purpose in attracting and arousing male humans— a crucial element in reproduction. It is the breasts that define our biological class: the word *mammal* comes from the term *mammary gland*—which is what the breast is. Despite the variance in mammals' breast size and number, mammals are the only biological group that breast*feeds*. But unlike other animals, human females develop full breasts long before they're needed for breastfeeding. This has to do with our sexual behavior, which makes it possible for us to engage in sex when we are not necessarily fertile. Nipple stimulation releases oxytocin, the hormone that not only triggers milk letdown but also uterine contractions, which researchers say enhances sexual sensation, particularly during orgasm.

Human breast tissue begins to develop in the sixth week of fetal life. The "milk ridge," a line from the armpit all the way down to the groin, develops at this point. In most cases, by the ninth week the milk ridge is in just the chest area, but both women and men can develop accessory nipples and even breast tissue all the way down to the groin. (These will look like moles to the untrained eye.) But other mammals retain the milk ridge, which is why they have multiple nipples. Therefore, when you're born, you already have breast tissue, as does your own newborn. And since the mother's sex hormones have been circulating through the placenta, both girls and boys are born with little breasts. Your newborn may even have milk production. This is known as "witch's milk," and it goes away in a couple of weeks, as the baby is weaned from your hormones. Between 80 and 90 percent of newborns may show some milk production the second or third day after birth.

For women, nothing much happens to the breast until puberty, when the pituitary gland starts the entire reproductive and development cycle. It is this kickstarting of the follicle-stimulating hormone (FSH)—which stimulates the ovary to produce estrogen, and then progesterone at ovulation—that triggers puberty. This includes the development of pubic hair, and so on. Young girls will usually sprout breast buds prior to pubic hair, but it could happen the other way around.

Breasts begin to develop at this point, and their development comprises five stages: the *prepubertal* stage, when the nipple becomes slightly more

Figure 1-1
ALVEOLUS (ENLARGED)

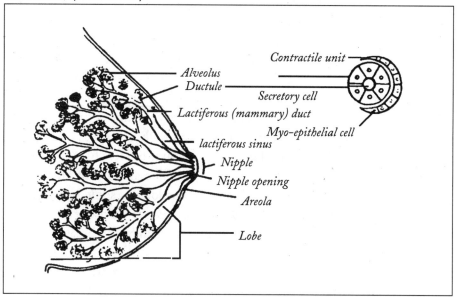

Source: The Breastfeeding Answer Book. *Reprinted with permission of La Leche League International, Inc., 1995.*

prominent; the *breast bud* stage, the beginning of breast growth; *breast elevation,* when the breast is formed and becomes more erect; the *areolar mound,* when the areola enlarges in circumference; and the *adult contour,* when the breast is mature enough to produce milk. The menstrual period is usually the "finale" to the breast's initial development. Further breast development occurs during pregnancy. This is currently the focus of extensive research, which may shed some light on why pregnancy (especially early pregnancy) tends to prevent breast cancer.

Breasts are considered mature when they are capable of producing milk, but the breast isn't considered fully *functional* until lactation actually begins. As you can see from figure 1-1, the breast is a gland considerably more complex than most women imagine.

Meet Your Mammary Gland

In the medical world, the breast is considered a "secretory gland" because it secretes fluids—in this case, milk. In order to produce milk, the breast relies on glandular tissue, which both produces and transports milk; connective tissue, which supports the breast so that it sits in an upright position; arterial blood supply, which not only nourishes breast tissue but delivers the essential nutrients to make milk; and the lymphatic system, which removes waste. (Lymph nodes, part of the lymphatic system, are like little POW camps that hold and "interrogate" foreign invaders.) The nerves in the breast are important elements in making the breast sensitive to the touch, thus allowing the baby's suckling to trigger the entire hormonal symphony responsible for milk production and milk letdown.

The breast is also comprised of a hefty amount of fatty tissue ("adipose tissue"), which protects the breast from injury. The amount of fatty tissue present determines the size of the breast, but as long as some breast tissue is present, *breast size has absolutely no effect on milk production or quality.* As long as the breasts begin to enlarge during pregnancy, the breasts are becoming fully functional.

Once milk production begins, things get a little more complicated. During lactation, the breast relies on *alveoli* (pronounced al-vee-oh-lie), grapelike clusters of glandular tissue that help to synthesize milk out of blood. Alveoli cells secrete milk and are surrounded by a layer of bandlike, myoepithelial cells that line them. If you imagine a real cluster of grapes, the myoepithelial cells are the grape skin, while the alveoli cells are the juicy pulp lying just beneath. When stimulated by oxytocin, the myoepithelial cells contract around the alveoli cells, which expel the milk into the ductules (see below) and into the milk ducts (also discussed below). For a simpler explanation, imagine a real grape between your fingers; when you squeeze the grape, it will squirt juice all over your hand. Continuing the analogy, oxytocin is the "squeeze" that makes the alveoli's milk squirt out.

The Transport System

Just like an automatic coffeemaker you may have at home, your breasts are fully equipped with a similar transport system that delivers the breast's liquids right down your baby's throat. Extending from the alveoli are branchlike tubes called *ductules.* Each of these ductules empties into larger ducts called *mammary ducts* (aka lactiferous ducts). Picture those real grape clusters again. Now imagine them still on the vine. The tiny branches leading to the stem would be the ductules, while the main stem connecting each grape cluster is the mammary duct. Each of these "stems" leads to the nipple.

Just before they reach the nipple, the mammary ducts swell and widen underneath the nipple and areola (the darker area of pigment surrounding the nipple) to become *lactiferous sinuses*. This is where the milk collects and waits for your baby to start suckling. The sinus narrows to an opening in the nipple (called a nipple pore). In fact, in order for these sinuses to be compressed and emptied, it's crucial that the nipple be fully in your baby's mouth, cradled between the tongue and palate, while the gums and lips should enclose most of the areola area. (This is more fully discussed in chapter 4.)

Going back to the grapevine analogy, several clusters of grapes will obviously be connected to a single stem. Well, within the breast, each of these "stems" forms a lobe. There are 15 to 25 lobes in the breast, and each lobe consists of 20 to 40 lobules (a smaller milk duct with its supporting alveoli). Each lobule, in turn, consists of 10 to 100 supporting alveoli. It's a little like that wooden Ukrainian doll game: Open up a lobe and you find within it a smaller, identical lobe; open up the smaller lobe, and you'll find a yet smaller one.

The Parts You Can Actually See

At last we come to the nipple. *All mammary ducts lead directly to the nipple.* After widening into a lactiferous sinus, the mammary duct narrows again and leads to the nipple opening, or pore. Some mammary ducts merge near the very tip of the nipple. Thanks to the delicate nerve endings, the nipple tissue is built to be extremely sensitive. When it's touched or stimulated, it protrudes and becomes firmer. It's also designed to be flexible and easily manipulated so it can fit the baby's mouth just right. Since each baby has differently shaped gums, palate, and tongue, the nipple needs to be moldable to any shape—including that of a cleft palate, which is discussed in chapter 8.

One of the most misunderstood parts of the breast is the areola, out of which the nipple protrudes. Many women become disturbed by the darkening of the areola during pregnancy, but there is a theory as to why it darkens. Your baby's eyesight takes several weeks to develop; at birth, then, the darkened areola serves as a "bull's eye target" to better allow for your newborn to find the center of the breast, where the nipple—and food—awaits. The darkened areola is also a signal for the baby to "suckle here, too," since, as we'll see further in chapter 4, successful breastfeeding depends on the areola being suckled as well. This is because the pattern of pressure and release of the baby's mouth on the *areola* stimulates the nerve pathways from the nipple to the brain to release the hormone prolactin into the bloodstream. Alveolar cells make milk in response to prolactin levels, which increase when the baby suckles at the breast. That's why things like nipple shields, a weak suckle, or improper positioning can alter prolactin levels and *cut down on milk supply!*

The areola also houses the Montgomery glands, which act as tiny muscles that contract and widen to help get the milk out. The Montgomery glands also produce oils that lubricate your nipple and discourage the growth of bacteria on the skin of the nipple and areola during lactation. The Montgomery glands enlarge during pregnancy, giving your areola that knobby appearance.

Understanding the importance of the Montgomery glands will also help reduce nipple irritation. For example, washing the nipples with soap is unnecessary and removes the beneficial oils that the Montgomery glands secrete. Such washing may also lead to drying and cracking, which can cause very sore nipples. (Sore nipples are discussed in detail in chapter 7.) To keep the nipples clean while preserving the essential lubricating oils and antibacterial properties that the Montgomery glands provide, just rinse your nipples with warm water while bathing.

The Pregnant and Postpartum Breast

The breasts are prepared for pregnancy each month. Estrogen causes the increase of ductal tissue in the breast, while progesterone causes the increase in lobular tissue. A common premenstrual symptom is swollen, sometimes painful breasts, which subside as the menstrual cycle comes to an end. But this common symptom can often be avoided with a simple adjustment in your diet (fat and caffeine are chief culprits) or even by lowering the estrogen content in your oral contraceptive dosage.

As discussed earlier, it is during pregnancy that the breasts enter their final stage of development and become, with the release of pregnancy hormones, fully functional. It's akin to blowing up a balloon. The balloon is ready anytime; all it needs is oxygen. Similarly, your breasts are ready to breastfeed by the time you get your first period; all they need is the hormonal burst, which then serves as their "oxygen."

Breast Changes

During pregnancy, when estrogen increases, it directly stimulates the ductules to grow, while progesterone's surge directly stimulates the alveoli and lobes to grow. Meanwhile, prolactin, discussed further below, causes all the surrounding tissues in the breast to grow. By the time you're five weeks pregnant, your breasts have already enlarged and become tender—something many women may first interpret as a premenstrual symptom. The breasts enlarge rapidly at this point and become firm. By around the seventh week, the Montgomery glands around the areola become darker and more prominent. The areola itself darkens even more, and the nipples become larger and more erect, preparing themselves for future milk production. By the tenth week of pregnancy, the breasts become large enough to warrant a good or just bigger support bra.

By the midpoint in your pregnancy, your breasts will have become fully functional, ready for breastfeeding. Around the twentieth week, your nipples may secrete a yellowish liquid, known as *colostrum*, a "premilk" discussed more below.

Breast changes during pregnancy vary from woman to woman. Most pregnant women experience breasts that swell, tingle, throb, or hurt. (Again, cutting out caffeine often helps.) Some women will notice early on that their nipples are very sensitive and sore. This is because the breast is developing milk glands. An increased blood supply going to the breasts causes the veins to become more pronounced, sometimes creating a network of enhanced blue lines under the skin around the breasts or abdomen. This is normal, due to the increased blood supply that is necessary to nourish the fetus.

Although immediately after delivery the breasts are ready for breastfeeding, as you'll read in later chapters, it takes some time for the breasts to develop mature milk. For the first few days of breastfeeding, an amazing substance called colostrum is produced, which nourishes the baby until the mature breast milk comes in. Colostrum contains complex immunological proteins, living white blood cells, and factors that activate bowel function. Colostrum not only keeps the customer satisfied until you begin producing mature milk, it helps to protect the baby from jaundice and many other infectious diseases. (See chapters 6 and 8 for more details.)

From the time of delivery until the actual milk comes in, the breast undergoes the most radical changes, and may become engorged with milk. *Engorgement can be prevented by beginning to breastfeed your baby colostrum immediately after childbirth and every two to three hours thereafter.* If a good start to breastfeeding is established at this juncture, you're well on the way to avoiding engorgement and the unnecessary pain and discomfort that so many women have suffered when starting to breastfeed. (Engorgement is discussed in great detail in chapter 7.)

The Milk Hormones

Two main hormones are responsible for milk production: prolactin and oxytocin (also responsible for triggering postpartum uterine contractions). Both these hormones are released by the pituitary gland, stimulated by an area of the brain known as the hypothalamus.

Prolactin is crucial for breastfeeding; without it, you don't make milk. Prolactin goes to work around the eighth week of pregnancy, and its levels rise for the next seven months, falling during the two to three hours prior to birth and peaking around three hours after delivery. During pregnancy, the body also produces high levels of estrogen and progesterone, which block some of the prolactin receptors and inhibit milk production. But once the baby is born, levels of estrogen and progesterone drop very quickly, while the prolactin levels follow at a far slower, almost unnoticeable rate. It is at this point that milk gets produced and breastfeeding can begin. If, for example, you choose not to breastfeed, the prolactin levels continue to drop and your breast milk dries up naturally. To keep up your prolactin levels and hence milk production, you must have nipple stimulation and you must empty your breasts.

Some researchers believe that together with oxytocin, prolactin, which is also called the "mothering hormone," may even be responsible for causing a mothering instinct to take root immediately after birth. This instinct translates into an intense desire on the mother's part to be with the baby, to cuddle the baby, and so on. This feeling of wanting to hold the baby close is actually part of the breastfeeding instinct that does come naturally. As you'll see in chapter 4, holding the baby close is one of the first steps involved when you begin to breastfeed.

Oxytocin, mentioned at the beginning of this chapter, is released during labor and anytime the nipple is stimulated. It's what makes your uterus "go." It contracts the smooth muscle of the uterus during labor and childbirth, after birth to help shrink the uterus back down to size, and during orgasm. In fact, to some women, the nipples feel like the "uterus switch." When you're breastfeeding, oxytocin also contracts the myoepithelial cells, which cause the alveoli to squeeze the newly produced milk out into the duct system. Oxytocin is crucial for what's called "milk letdown" or the "milk-ejection reflex." Milk letdown makes the milk available to the baby—particularly the fatty, creamier hindmilk, which the baby needs to feel satisfied. (Hindmilk is discussed more in chapters 6 and 8.) When the baby is latched on properly to the breast, the suckling stimulates the nerve endings in the nipple (via thoracic nerves) and areola, signaling your pituitary gland to send down more milk. When the pituitary gland gets this message, it first releases oxytocin and then prolactin into the bloodstream. (Chapter 4 discusses milk letdown in more detail.)

Supply and Demand

All of your breasts' parts and hormones work on a clever supply-and-demand schedule. The baby's suckling, as discussed above, not only sends a message to the pituitary gland to make more oxytocin but also calls for more prolactin, which gradually increases the amount of milk that is made. The suckling triggers more milk; the lack of regular suckling inhibits milk production. An inadequate milk supply almost always has more to do with ineffective breastfeeding than with a physical inability to produce enough milk.

Quite simply, the baby's suckling controls the amount of milk you produce. And so your milk supply will dwindle if you're separated from your baby and do not express/pump your breasts to replace feedings (see chapter 5); you place your baby on a strict feeding schedule (fully exposed as a no-no in chapter 4); you substitute other liquids or solids for breastfeeding; you delay breastfeeding or breastfeed infrequently. The good news is that the breast milk supply is highly resilient; even under these circumstances it can often be built up again, in anything from a few days to a few weeks.

The Second-Oldest Profession

Wet-nursing is such an old profession that French archaeologists found the tomb of Tutankhamen's wet nurse. The supply-and-demand principle of breastfeeding is so reliable that it has helped to feed many more mouths than just babies'.

In the days when wet nurses existed, aristocratic mothers would not breastfeed because they were considered too frail to produce "good milk." Instead, a wet nurse would be engaged. Wet nurses stayed "wet" by continually breastfeeding after they themselves had children. In effect, one could—and still can—conceivably breastfeed for years; so long as the suckling was there, the breast milk would continue to some extent.

Wet-nursing became so popular between the 17th and mid-19th centuries that many young girls would deliberately have illegitimate children and then send them to "baby farms" in the country (where most of them died), so that they could be easily employed. Many established wet nurses would get pregnant again just to increase milk supply and promote their employability (also abandoning their own babies). When wet nurses were not available, "dry nursing," now called relactation (see chapter 5), would be attempted.

Thought Control

As you may already know, your own thoughts can influence your milk letdown. Merely thinking about your baby, hearing your baby, or smelling your baby can trigger the pituitary's release of oxytocin into the bloodstream and set the letdown reflex in motion.

In contrast, strong emotions such as anger or sadness can inhibit milk letdown. The influence of our emotions on our hormones is not, however, entirely surprising. Menstrual cycles are highly vulnerable to external stresses, too. For this reason, lactation consultants are all too aware that one's emotional mind-set can have either positive or negative effects on lactation hormones. For example, a mother who is feeling anxious, insecure, or extremely fatigued and lethargic after childbirth may have more difficulty with milk letdown. In the same way that stress can prevent ovulation, it can also inhibit oxytocin. Nurses and midwives report that when new mothers are having difficulty with milk letdown, reassurance, emotional support, and a little rest and relaxation are often the remedies. (This is discussed further in chapter 4.)

THE TROUBLE WITH NIPPLES

Any part of our body can be vulnerable to slight anatomical variations. The breast is no exception. In our culture, small-breasted women and large-breasted women often see their breasts as "abnormal" or defective because of a size they view as "unproportional." For the record, breasts come in all sizes, and no size is considered clinically abnormal. What a breast *does* need to produce milk is breast glandular tissue. In rare cases, women may have a breast made up of just skin and a nipple, or else breast fat without any breast glandular tissue. These women would not be able to produce milk. But so long as your breasts have increased in size during pregnancy *or* after birth, and if you felt slight breast tenderness during pregnancy, you're fine.

More common problems have to do with nipple engineering. In a woman who isn't breastfeeding, these nipple variations are harmless and do not significantly influence her lifestyle. But for a woman planning to breast-feed, some nipple variations may pose a problem.

The two most common nipple variations are *flat nipples*, where the nipple does not become erect when stimulated or cold, and *inverted nipples*, where the nipples retract into the breast rather than protrude when the areola is compressed. Some women may have one normal nipple and one flat or inverted nipple. Others may have one flat nipple, with the other one inverted.

Breast size has nothing to do with nipple architecture. And as stated earlier on, breast size has absolutely nothing to do with milk supply. Some small-breasted women may produce copious amounts of milk, while other large-breasted women may have to express/pump their breasts between feedings just to manufacture enough milk. Sore nipples, one of the key breastfeeding beefs, is discussed in chapter 7.

Flat Nipples

A nipple is truly "flat" when there is no way to make it erect. It will not respond to cold, sexual stimulation, or a baby's suckling.

In some women, engorgement can cause *temporary* flat nipples, which will subside after breastfeeding continues for a few days. (If you haven't delivered yet, I'll tell you how to prevent engorgement altogether in chapters 3 and 4.) In other women, nipples are congenitally (meaning "present from birth") flat.

Breastfeeding with flat nipples is a lot easier if you've prepared a little ahead of time. A variety of methods are available that will "draw out" nipples so that you can breastfeed comfortably. Treating flat nipples and preparing them for breastfeeding are discussed in chapter 3. Latching techniques that work with flat nipples are discussed in chapter 4. Breast shells, discussed below and in chapter 3, were once thought to help, but recent research has exposed them to be useless.

Inverted Nipples

Imagine the tip of a condom. Now take your pinky finger and poke the tip inward so that it lies *inside* the condom. That's what an inverted nipple will do when you squeeze the areola. Many women don't realize their nipples are inverted until they begin to breastfeed, because an inverted nipple may look like a normal nipple; it just won't act like one!

Inverted nipples are extremely easy to treat by drawing them out with a few manual tricks I'll discuss in chapter 3. Traditionally, breast shells (which look like a rubber or plastic areola with a hole in the center out of which your nipple pokes), were the treatment of choice by lactation practitioners. They were designed to be worn between feedings to supposedly train the nipple to poke out normally. So why didn't they work? Unfortunately, such things (also referred to as breast shields, milk cups, breast cups, or Woolwich shields) can make you more prone to infections, which can interfere with breastfeeding. (They are discussed in the Booby Traps section in chapter 3.)

Don't confuse breast shells with nipple shields, also a horrible product but designed to be worn over the nipple and areola during feeding to reduce soreness. Nipple shields are also discussed in chapter 3.

The Combo Platter

Even if you have one normal nipple (which becomes erect easily), and one flat or inverted nipple, you still need to be prepared to help your baby latch onto it so that you can empty both breasts, or else you will suffer from engorgement and discomfort. As we'll discuss in chapter 4, each breast must be emptied *separately*; there is no "tunnel" that links one breast to the other, allowing the milk to flow easily from left breast to right. Each mammary gland, in other words, functions as a separate entity. One-sided nursing (discussed in chapter 8) is possible, however, if you express the other breast manually (discussed in chapter 5).

THINGS THAT GO WRONG INSIDE THE BREAST

Because your breasts are a complex system of ducts and lobes, they can become clogged by inflammations, abscesses, or even lumps. This can create problems with your milk supply and may cause breast pain, a sign that something's wrong. Breast pain is never "just one of those things." When your breasts hurt, there's usually a good reason. Breast pain and breast infections are thoroughly covered in chapter 7. Women who are prone to breast cysts and breast lumps can usually breastfeed without difficulty, as we'll discuss in chapter 2.

If your milk supply is dwindling or isn't establishing itself, the problem is less likely to lie with the breast itself than with your hormones. A hormonal deficiency may be blocking the MAKE MILK messages your pituitary gland should be receiving. For the record, however, less than 1 percent of the entire female population suffers from a lagging milk supply due to hormonal imbalance. The majority of lagging milk supplies are due to a *bad latch*, something we'll discuss more fully in chapter 4.

If you *do* happen to be in the minority, and despite a good latch and good breastfeeding management you still cannot make milk, your doctor can prescribe *lactagogues*, hormonal supplements that will signal your pituitary gland to tell your breasts to make milk. Lactagogues are discussed in chapters 4, 6, and 7.

Doctor-Made Breast Problems

Since we are currently living in a time when one in nine women develops breast cancer and many first-time mothers are over thirty-five, there will no doubt be many women attempting to breastfeed after breast cancer surgery who may even have had reconstructive surgery or breast implants.

And since the breasts are sexual objects in our society that can make or break a woman's self-esteem, many women have undergone breast reduction surgery or breast augmentation surgery employing breast implants. If you are one of these women, please read chapter 2. Some of you may be able to breastfeed beautifully, but many of you may experience problems due to scar tissue inside the breast that blocks milk ducts or even interferes with the alveoli.

BSE: Breast Self-Examination

In 1995, every woman over thirty should be aware that she's living through a breast cancer epidemic, due in part to the fact that not enough women breastfeed (which reduces the risk of breast cancer). So if you've never performed BSE before, get into the habit today. Now. BSE is not about finding breast cancer; it's about getting to know your breasts. Whether you're breastfeeding or not, your pregnancy has brought about *tremendous* changes in your breasts. Unless you know what your breasts normally feel like, and which lumps and bumps are just you and which are not, you won't be able to recognize a suspicious breast lump.

BSE involves a specific routine of feeling your breast at around the same time each month (preferably just after you've menstruated). That way you may be able to distinguish suspicious lumps from milk cysts, enlarged lymph nodes, and so on. In addition, you can't know if a lump is suspicious and has remained "unchanged" unless you've been checking your breasts regularly. While ideally you should begin BSE by the age of twenty, starting now—however old you are—is just fine. When breastfeeding, perform BSE on a monthly basis after feeding, when your breasts aren't filled with milk. When your menstrual cycle returns, the BSE will be most effective right after your period, when your baby has just fed. It's at this time that your breasts are least tender and lumpy and you won't be mistaking PMS tenderness and lumpiness for anything suspicious. Make sure your doctor goes over the following steps with you:

1. *Visually inspect your breasts.* Stand in front of the mirror and look closely at your breasts. You're looking for dimpling, puckering (like an orange peel in appearance), or noticeable lumps (which you can't often see). Do you see any unusual discharge that dribbles out on its own or bleeding from the nipple? Any funny dry patches on the nipple (which may be Paget's disease)?

2. *Visually inspect your breasts with your arms raised.* Now, still in front of the mirror, raise your arms over your head and look for the same things. Raising your arms smoothes out the breast a little more so that these changes are more obvious.

3. *Palpation (feeling your breast).* Lie down on your bed with a pillow under your left shoulder and place your left hand under your head. With the flat part of the fingertips of your right hand, examine your left breast for a lump, using a gentle circular motion. Imagine that the breast is a clock, and make sure you feel each "hour," as well as the nipple area and armpit area.

4. *Repeat step 3, but reverse sides, examining your right breast with your left hand.*

5. *If you find a lump . . . note the size, shape, and how painless it is.* A suspicious lump is usually painless, about ¼–½ inch in size, and remains unchanged from month to month. Get your lump looked at as soon

as you can, or if you're comfortable doing so, wait for one month. If the lump changes in the next month by shrinking or becoming painful, it's not cancerous but should be looked at anyway. If the suspicious lump stays the same, definitely get it looked at as soon as possible. Keep in mind that breast cysts are common, variable in size, and occasionally tender.

6. *If discharge other than breast milk oozes out of your nipple on its own, or if blood comes out . . .* see your doctor immediately. Don't wait.

7. *If your nipple is dry and patchy . . . see your doctor immediately.* Don't wait.

For the record, 90 percent of all breast cancers are picked up by women themselves, either accidentally or through BSE. At all times of your life (particularly when your breasts are continually changing as a result of pregnancy and breastfeeding), BSE should become a monthly ritual. As you wean and your breasts decrease in fullness, or perhaps prepare for yet another pregnancy, breast changes will mean that you need to constantly familiarize yourself with them. If you haven't delivered yet or are planning another child, *continue your BSE throughout all stages of your pregnancy. You can get breast cancer while you're pregnant.*

৵৯

Congratulations, you just passed the anatomy course! Now that you know where milk comes from, it's time to make a decision about how you'll feed your child. The next chapter is designed to answer all those questions and doubts you have about breastfeeding. How much time and money do you really save? What are the nutritional issues of breastfeeding vs. formula feeding? Are there any environmental dangers you should know about?

Whether you're diabetic, wear silicone breast implants, are taking any medications, are so confused about the breastfeeding literature you don't know *what* to believe, or just can't seem to picture yourself breastfeeding, chapter 2 will help you make the decision so you can plan for the best feeding experience possible.

Since for a few of you breastfeeding may *not* be the best decision after all, the next chapter will also discuss all the alternatives to breastfeeding.

chapter 2

$\mathcal{M}$AKING THE $\mathcal{D}$ECISION

*I*f you're confused about breastfeeding, it's understandable. The problem with making the "breastfeeding decision" is that breastfeeding shouldn't have to be positioned as a decision or a choice in the first place. Breastfeeding is the normal way for a female mammal to feed her baby. It is not a woman's choice, but her right. Feeding your baby milk that is not your own is not a normal thing for our species to do. But in cases where breastfeeding or breast milk is not at all possible, and there is no other alternative, artificial baby milk or formula will have to do.

Artificial baby milk was a product originally designed as a last resort. It was never intended for routine use, though some women need to feed their babies artificial milk because of various health conditions. As I explain in chapter 11, breastfeeding was transformed from a woman's right to a "decision" or "choice" through baby formula marketing.

BREASTFEEDING MYTHOLOGY

It's estimated that prior to delivery, between 80 and 90 percent of all pregnant women want to breastfeed. After delivery, unless there's emotional support, adequate training, and information about *how* to breastfeed, some of these women just give up. According to many public-health nurses and lactation consultants, one of the most influential forces in the breastfeeding decision is your own mother: your baby's grandmother. If she didn't breastfeed ("I bottlefed *all* of my children and you turned out just fine!" "Trust me, once you start, you'll be chained to the house. What about your husband and *career?*"), you can expect some resistance, subtle or overt. *But you don't have to let it determine your own decision.* Respond with "But don't you want what's best for me and the baby? All doctors agree that breastfeeding is not only superior to formula but protects me against breast cancer." (You might also remind Mom that one in nine women now get breast cancer.) Why would your own mother—of all people—undermine your breastfeeding decision? The answer is simple: guilt. Women who bottle-fed in the past often feel guilty about not having breastfed. *And many of these same women smoked and drank during pregnancy too.* The bottom line is that hindsight is 20/20. We simply know more today about what's best for baby than we did thirty or even twenty years ago. So if you want to breastfeed but are being discouraged by older family matriarchs, keep in mind that it is an *undisputed* medical fact that "breast is best" for baby and you, physically and emotionally.

The Feeding Frenzy

Most of the myths regarding breastfeeding are rooted in gossip feeding frenzies. Here are some common myths:

Myth: If you have your first baby when you're over thirty-five, your breast milk won't be as nutritious.
Fact: Having a first child late in life will not affect your breast milk *at all.* You'll be able to produce milk that's as good at forty as you would have at twenty.

Myth: You can't get pregnant while you're breastfeeding.
Fact: Breastfeeding has been touted as being a natural contraceptive, but it's not 100 percent effective. This is discussed more in chapter 10.

Myth: You have to stop breastfeeding if you're going back to work.
Fact: Nonsense! If you're going back to work, you can express/pump your breasts every three or four hours for milk and cool and refrigerate it to use the next day, or else freeze it. (Chapters 5 and 9 address these issues.)

Myth: There's nothing you can do about sore nipples when you're breastfeeding; you just have to live with it.
Fact: Wrong again! Air and using your own milk as an anti-infective agent can work wonders, as well as learning the proper feeding technique to begin

with. But even in extreme cases, avoid rubber nipple shields; these will interfere with lactation and may confuse the baby. Under these circumstances, see a lactation consultant about your positioning.

Myth: You can't breastfeed if you have inverted nipples.
Fact: Review chapter 1 if you're unsure what is meant by "inverted nipples." In any case, you can breastfeed with inverted nipples. You'll find out how in chapter 3.

Myth: You can't breastfeed if you have breast cancer or were treated for breast cancer.
Fact: You *can* breastfeed out of a cancerous breast. Your child will not "catch" breast cancer, and the milk will be just as good and nutritious. But if you're currently undergoing chemotherapy or hormonal therapy, you cannot breastfeed. See the Women in Special Circumstances section further on.

Myth: Breastfeeding with breasts with silicone implants is perfectly safe, posing no risk to your child.
Fact: This is still being debated. You can technically breastfeed out of breasts with implants, but there have been reports of health problems in children who were fed from breasts with implants. Worse, women with older implants are themselves reporting alarming health problems, which would further indicate proceeding with caution. (Again, see Women in Special Circumstances section for more details.)

Myth: There is no documented proof that HIV is transmitted through breast milk. If you're HIV positive, it's still better to breastfeed than to risk formula.
Fact: There is *plenty* of documented proof that HIV can be passed from a mother to child through breast milk. Every woman has the right to confidential HIV testing.

Myth: Bottle-fed babies don't bond with their mothers, which is why it's imperative to breastfeed.
Fact: Bonding has more to do with loving, holding, and nurturing your baby and providing a loving environment. If you are one of the few who should not breastfeed, bottle-feeding should be a guilt-free choice.

Myth: Nipples must be "toughened up" in advance before you begin to breastfeed.

Fact: No, they don't! If your nipples are normal (i.e., not flat or inverted) and the baby has a good latch, they need no advance preparation.

Myth: Blondes have more pain; fair-haired and fair-skinned breastfeeders will have sorer nipples than darker-haired or darker-skinned mothers.
Fact: Utter nonsense. Sore nipples result from a bad latch or position. (Chapters 4 and 7 further explore this subject.)

Myth: Unless you feed your baby immediately after birth, you're doomed to have a bad experience.
Fact: It is ideal to feed within the *first couple of hours after birth*. But even if you do miss the opportunity, there's plenty of time to rectify the situation.

WHAT'S IN IT FOR BABY?

Your breast milk *changes* continuously to meet the needs of your baby. For example, toward the end of a feeding, a "hindmilk" is produced, which contains more fat, giving the baby a sense of fullness and satisfaction. In climate changes, the milk adapts amazingly well, containing more water in hot weather and more calories in cold weather, to keep up the baby's energy. During your baby's growth spurts, breast milk will also provide more proteins, fats, and calories.

Your baby can also digest breast milk more easily, breaking down the proteins, fats, and sugars much more efficiently than with formula. Breast milk also contains less sodium and protein, which puts less stress on your baby's kidneys. Furthermore, it allows the baby to better absorb calcium and increases protection against several infections that can affect the lungs, ears, bladder, stomach, and bowel. Breast milk has been known as well to help prevent diabetes, sudden infant death syndrome (SIDS), childhood cancer, and Chron's disease.

Breastfed babies suffer far less from allergies, constipation, diarrhea, and diaper rash. Interestingly, breastfed babies also smell sweeter than bottle-fed babies. New studies also demonstrate that breastfeeding offers protection against acute respiratory infections, lower respiratory tract infections, middle ear infections, and bacterial meningitis.

It's been found that breastfed babies are generally less obese later in life (some studies estimate that bottle-fed babies are *four times* more likely to become obese), because breastfed babies stop feeding when they're full, while bottle-fed babies are encouraged to overstuff themselves. There is also lower cholesterol in breastfed babies, better mouth development, and fewer cavities and orthodontic problems.

The World Health Organization now recommends that breastfeeding be continued until at least two years of age. This translates into fully breastfeeding (breast milk only) for the first four to six months of age, then supplementing breast milk with solid foods until a year of age, then using breast milk as a supplement until two years of age. New Zealand researchers who followed 1,000 children since 1977 recently concluded that breastfeeding is associated with small but detectable increases in cognitive ability and educational achievement.

The Ingredients

The reason why formula companies position their product as "most like mother's milk" is because it's impossible to exactly duplicate the nutrients. In fact, most health experts point out that there's really no formula that comes even close to breast milk in terms of nutrition.

In an age where we can "grow" human beings in a test tube, what is it about human breast milk that is so miraculous it can't be synthetically reproduced? Breast milk is what scientists refer to as "species specific." Human milk, like other mammals' milk, adapts itself to meet the exact nutritional requirements of the human baby. And it does so in some very precise ways.

Exact Quantity

A healthy lactating woman won't have to worry about leftovers unless she's expressing or pumping her milk. That's because of the supply-and-demand hormonal system discussed in chapter 1. For example, during the baby's first month of feeding, the breasts will produce roughly 600 ml of milk for the baby, progress to about 700–750 ml per day when the baby's three months old, and finally reach about 800 ml per day by the baby's sixth month. At that point, the breast milk supply will start to decline in volume as the baby's diet begins to include other liquids, as well as solids. Each 100 ml of human milk is equal to about 75 calories of energy, on average, depending upon the baby's sex, genes, and growth pattern.

High in Saturated Fats

The one thing you can't say about breast milk is that it's low-fat. In fact, one of the most important ingredients in breast milk is fat. But incredibly (researchers are still trying to figure out why it does this), the fat content changes, depending upon the time of day. It's lowest at 6 A.M. and peaks at about 2 P.M. As discussed in chapter 1, most of the fat is contained in the hindmilk, which is made available to the baby through oxytocin, causing milk letdown.

Human milk contains the enzyme lipase, which is also found in the breastfed baby's intestine. Lipase is important because it breaks down the fat from triglycerides (the basic ingredient of all fat) into fatty acids and glycerol. What happens in breast milk, though, is that the baby never gets a mouthful of triglycerides, but an already digested, broken-down form of the fat, which the baby experiences as a steady, smooth flow of energy. The protein is more digestible too, because it doesn't "clump."

Goes Down Smooth

Prostaglandins is another ingredient in breast milk. During menstruation, prostaglandins, a chemical secreted by our tissues, is what pushes out our uterine lining each month. So what on earth is it doing in breast milk? That's something researchers are still trying to figure out, but it's now known that it helps the baby's digestive tract move more smoothly. In other words, researchers believe its what makes the baby's digestive tract "go."

As for lactose, it's in all mammal milk, but there seems to be more of it in human milk. The condition known as lactose intolerance stems from not having the enzyme lactase in your system, which breaks down lactose into simple sugars, necessary for digestion. Babies are born with lactase in their intestinal systems, and only in very rare cases do they not have the enzyme. But as the baby grows, the enzyme can get "used up," creating lactose intolerance in later life. Most people who are lactose intolerant seem to have a problem only with digesting lactose from cow's milk, and not goat's milk or human milk. Lactose is responsible for providing human milk with carbohydrates. (See chapter 8 for more information on infant lactose intolerance.)

Whey to Go

In terms of protein, cow's milk actually has more of it than human milk. Whey and casein are the main sources of protein in all milk. Human milk has more whey than cow's milk does, however, which makes it more digestible for a baby. Casein breaks down into a more rubbery consistency and tends to just sit in the baby's stomach, requiring a lot more energy on the baby's part to digest it.

Extras

There are also two important amino acids in breast milk that are not in cow's milk: cystine and taurine, essential to the baby's brain development. Breast milk also contains DHA (docosahexaenoic acid), an essential fatty acid largely responsible for eye and brain development. As a result of this finding, the World Health Organization has recommended that DHA be included in infant formulas. Meanwhile, colostrum, the "premilk" substance discussed in chapter 1, contains ten essential amino acids and has three times the protein of mature breast milk.

Vitamins and Minerals

Generally, as long as your own diet is healthy, your baby is getting the right amount of vitamins and minerals. Human breast milk is particularly high in vitamin C, while colostrum is very high in vitamin E. Human milk, like cow's milk, is very high in zinc; only human milk, however, has a zinc-binding action that helps the baby absorb it better.

It might surprise you to learn that breast milk has very little iron (only 0.5 to 1 mg per liter), but as long as you both are healthy and your pregnancy diet was nutritious, your baby won't need any additional iron before six months. After that, solids will begin, supplying the necessary iron levels. Moreover, because breast milk contains such high levels of lactose and vitamin C, the small amount of iron breast milk does contain is absorbed completely. Formula-fed babies need more iron, because formula makes the bowels bleed slightly, causing iron loss that must be compensated for.

Low in Salt

Breast milk has lower levels of calcium, phosphorus, sodium, and potassium than cow's milk has. That boils down to less salt, which means less stress on the kidneys and not as much thirst as a baby drinking formula or cow's milk develops. It also means that the breastfed baby is more able to tolerate and recover from illnesses like diarrhea without becoming as dehydrated as a formula-fed baby.

The Anti-Infective Properties

Among the most highly regarded aspects of breast milk are its anti-infective properties. Both colostrum and breast milk contain loads of enzymes, immunoglobulins, and white blood cells—all anti-infective agents. An example of how jam-packed breast milk is with this stuff: the enzyme lysozyme, also present in cow's milk, is about 5,000 times more concentrated in breast milk.

Antiallergic Properties

Because breast milk doesn't have the classic ingredients that tend to cause food allergies and stomach upset, it's said to be "antiallergic." Moreover, breast milk is as fresh as you can get it and doesn't involve any heating or transporting. (See chapter 8 for more information on allergies.)

WHAT'S IN IT FOR YOU?

Breast milk is more nutritious; it's always the right temperature; you can breastfeed while you doze; it's cheap; it's convenient and safe; it's instant, fast food; it's available for as long as you need it; it helps your uterus shrink; it helps you lose weight—particularly in the thighs; and it helps you bond. With the aid of breast pumps, working mothers can breastfeed and other family members can help with feedings.

Yet in addition to all the above, a further compelling reason to choose breastfeeding is that it offers protection against breast and ovarian cancer. Because breastfeeding delays the ovulation cycle a little longer than pregnancy alone, this gives your ovaries a nice vacation—something that most cancerous ovaries don't get. The ovaries also make estrogen, which may encourage breast cancer cells to grow. Give the ovaries a break from making follicles (eggs) and estrogen, and you greatly reduce the risk of estrogen-dependent cancers, such as those associated with the breast and ovaries.

Researchers at the University of Buffalo found that women with breast cancer who had never breastfed had significantly higher levels of organochlorines in their blood than healthy women who had breastfed their infants. It's believed that these chemicals are stored in fatty tissue, such as breast tissue, and that breastfeeding helps to flush these toxins from the system.

Many women have expressed concern, however, about exposing their babies to organochlorines through breast milk. But, experts maintain that breastfeeding remains the best way to feed your baby.

Will I Have Any Time to Myself?

No, not at first. But that's true no matter *how* you feed your baby. Breastfeeding may require some learning time up front, but once you get the hang of it, it saves you much more time later on. You can also be as mobile as you like; just take the baby with you and breastfeed wherever you are. You don't need bottles, formula, a place to heat the bottles, and so on.

One of the most common reasons for early weaning has to do with the "no time to myself" issue. If you've read elsewhere that breastfeeding is not all that time-consuming, *it's a lie*. But with a little help from your friends or breastfeeding buddies in a peer-support group, and the right support from a qualified lactation consultant, you'll get used to the fact that when you have a baby, regardless of feeding method, your time is *not* your own anymore. That's largely what parenting involves, anyway. Just ask your *own* mother! We discuss issues involving time in later chapters. And there are ways to maximize the little time you do have left to yourself!

ABOUT YOUR FOOD AND DRUGS

For many women, one of the most influential factors in the breastfeeding decision revolves around what you can and cannot eat, drink, and smoke.

Yet over-the-counter and prescription drugs may affect breast milk—and hence your baby—even more than a junk-food diet.

What to Eat

Throw out all those articles and books preaching puritanical diets during breastfeeding! Growing your own organic food and drinking a gallon of homemade carrot juice every day may be ideal if you live on a farm, but it's not very practical when you live in an urban setting, and particularly when caring for a newborn. (All that carotene would turn both you and the baby orange, too.)

Traditional, calorie-grounded thinking held that breastfeeding mothers needed to take in 500 additional calories per baby *per day* above their prepregnancy calorie intake. So, one baby = 500 extra calories; 2 babies = 1,000; 3 babies = 1,500; and so on. This extra 500 calories per baby per day was 500 calories above your prepregnancy calorie intake! Now research suggests that the extra-500-calorie-per-baby-per-day allowance may be too high. So the best advice, according to lactation consultants, is this: *Eat when you're hungry, and eat good stuff!*

If you're concerned about quality control, consult a nutritionist (ask your doctor for recommendations) about your normal diet routine. Some helpful nutrition tips include sticking to mostly the outside aisles of a supermarket when food shopping, reading labels, and avoiding anything that comes out of a can. Many doctors simply advise that if you find that a label has words you can't pronounce or never heard of, ask a nutritionist or doctor before you eat it. And as for canned foods, even those may get a reprieve: It's been found that if you rinse the salt off many canned vegetables, they end up with even higher vitamin levels than their fresh counterparts.

Perhaps the most important advice regarding your diet is *don't crash diet*—particularly when you breastfeed. Sudden weight loss will not only affect your milk supply but your overall health. Losing weight too quickly may also cause you to release environmental contaminants into your milk, which are normally stored in body fat. Since your body will instinctively tap into your "baby fat" (your pregnancy weight) and use it as fuel for milk production anyway, there's no need to starve or purge yourself.

On the flip side, there are no magical foods you can eat that will increase milk supply, either. If you want to take vitamin supplements, that's fine, but a vitamin supplement cannot replace a good, commonsense diet.

The average weight loss during the first six months of breastfeeding is about two pounds per month. If you're losing more than four pounds per month, this is considered too much too fast for lactation. To keep your weight loss gradual, snacking between meals really helps.

Finally, not all women lose weight during breastfeeding. If you're not losing your weight, you may not *need* to lose any weight, or else your body may need to put *on* weight. Other women find that weight comes off toward the end of breastfeeding, or even after weaning. If you're worried, consult a nutritionist to tailor your diet accordingly.

Drink When You're Thirsty

All nutritionists will tell you to drink enough fluids to prevent constipation and dehydration. Since women come in all shapes and sizes, however, adhering to a strict amount (such as eight glasses of water per day) isn't necessary. In fact, forcing down more fluids than you feel like drinking will make you uncomfortable.

As a rule, if your urine is pale yellow, you're getting enough fluids. If you're constipated and/or your urine is a darker shade of yellow, with a strong smell, this is a sign that you should drink more fluids. What constitutes "fluid" other than water? Fresh fruits and vegetables, soups, fruit juices, and milk.

Taste Tests

Garlic lovers and chocoholics, beware! Strong flavors and spices may affect your breast milk and may not agree with your baby. Classic newborn irritants include: garlic, onion, cabbage (gas), and anything with cow's milk (causing colic).

You'll have to test and see. Many women find, for example, that after a Szechuan pig-out session their baby's digestive system reacts negatively to their milk. If, however, your baby doesn't mind your spices and choices, there's no reason to cut them out.

Chocolate, caffeine, and sugar can cause your newborn to be fussy, but most babies are unaffected by even five cups (not mugs) of coffee per day and less than a pound of chocolate a day. As for sugar, use your judgment. The general rule for caffeine is that if you consume the equivalent of five or more cups of coffee per day, your baby may become stimulated by it too. When you're caffeine-counting, however, don't forget iced and hot tea, colas, and even over-the-drugs that contain caffeine. Chocolate, by the way, does *not* contain caffeine, but a substance known as theobromine, which is very similar to caffeine and acts as a stimulant. Modest amounts of chocolate are usually not significant, but just like adults, some babies are more sensitive to it than others. (Chapter 8 discusses food irritants in more detail.)

Don'ts and Nevers

You probably know all these by heart by now, but all of the "don'ts and nevers" you practiced during pregnancy regarding smoking, alcohol, and narcotics apply here as well. Whether it's your placenta or your breast, your baby is still affected by what you're drinking, smoking, or injecting.

Smoking is *always* a bad idea—particularly when you breastfeed. Smoking can significantly reduce your prolactin levels, which may affect your milk supply. If you absolutely cannot stop smoking while breastfeeding, try to cut down your habit by *at least* half. Also try to time your smoking so that it takes place at least one hour after breastfeeding; nicotine lowers breast-milk production.

According to many lactation experts, if you smoke fewer than twenty cigarettes per day, the amount of nicotine in your milk (roughly 0.5) will probably not affect your baby, but the American Academy of Pediatrics lists any amount of nicotine as "contraindicated" (i.e., harmful) during breastfeeding. Recently, Canadian researchers found extremely high levels of cotinine (what nicotine becomes when it is broken down in the body) in infants who were breastfed by mothers who also smoke. These levels were almost as high as in an adult who smokes nearly twenty cigarettes a day. Too much nicotine can cause shock, vomiting, diarrhea, rapid heart rate, and restlessness. If you can't stop smoking, weigh the risks of your smoking against the risk of not breastfeeding.

If you choose to smoke and breastfeed, and you're having difficulty with your milk supply because of reduced prolactin levels, you'll need to choose between smoking or breastfeeding. A lactogogue might be administered to get your milk supply up, but you'd be much better off just quitting. Remember, too, that secondhand smoke is perhaps even *more* damaging to your baby than nicotine levels in breast milk. Myriad studies conclude that yes, babies who breathe in smoke from one or both parents don't feel as well as babies born to nonsmokers. If you don't mind increasing your baby's risk of developing pneumonia, bronchitis, or even SIDS (sudden infant death syndrome), then there's no reason to quit. Studies show that children between two to twenty-four months, who were exposed to cigarette smoke, were more likely to have asthma, chronic bronchitis, and a history of wheezing than unexposed children. In fact, researchers found that up to 60 percent of all asthma, chronic bronchitis, and three or more episodes of wheezing were directly caused by exposure to smoke.

As for alcohol, it takes about thirty minutes for the alcohol you consume to reach your milk. A glass of wine or beer with dinner won't affect your breastfeeding, but large amounts of alcohol can affect your oxytocin levels, which inhibit your milk letdown. If you are a heavy drinker, not only will *you* suffer all the ill effects of alcohol abuse, but your baby will become intoxicated too. She may sleep through feedings, not be able to suck as strongly, and will therefore not thrive. Brain development will also be affected. If you're breastfeeding, drink alcohol judiciously or not at all.

Any drug that is illegal is always bad news—worse news when you're pregnant or breastfeeding. (See the separate section on illegal drugs on page 30 for more details. Prescription and over-the-counter drugs are covered in separate sections on pages 31 to 33.)

A Word to Low-Income Mothers

As discussed at the beginning of this chapter, many doctors traditionally counseled low-income women against breastfeeding, believing that an unbalanced diet would affect the breast milk's nutrients. *This is not true.* When it comes to just plain food in North America, even the poorest diets do not affect breast milk whatsoever. Only mothers who are chronically and severely malnourished have reduced milk supplies. And in order to fall into that category, you'd have to live in a country like Somalia!

It's also much less expensive to buy nutritious food than formula. If you're tempted by formula companies with a free case of formula delivered to you, the director of the Breastfeeding Clinic at Toronto's Hospital for Sick Children advises that it's better to use that free formula in your baked goods than to give it to your baby. That way, *you'll* get the nutrients that the formula contains, which will help boost your diet for breastfeeding. And you won't waste the formula. (Hint: Substitute formula in any recipe that calls for milk or condensed milk.)

Avoiding Environmental Toxins

Since Earth is a pretty toxic planet, nutritionists may not be as indispensable to breastfeeding mothers as environmentalists!

You'll want to make sure that your fruits and veggies are washed well to help eliminate pesticides from your diet, and you may want to rethink eating that trout from your brother-in-law's fishing trip. Any fish or seafood bought in a large supermarket chain is inspected, and therefore considered safe. Obviously, less-processed, more natural foods are better. To find out where to buy the safest food and what to avoid, Americans can contact the Public Information Center of the Environmental Protection Agency at (202) 382-2080 or the Food Safety and Inspection Service at (202) 447-9351. Canadians can contact the Ministry or Department of Environment, listed provincially, or Environment Canada (at the federal level) at (613) 997-2800.

Finally, investigate whether there are any nuclear or chemical plants in your area. Breathing contaminated air, drinking contaminated water, and eating pesticide-free food from contaminated soil is worse news in pregnancy but still bad news when breastfeeding. Just make sure you know what you're eating and breathing. Review the tables of workplace hazards and their effects on reproductive organs in chapter 9.

Illegal Drugs

If you're breastfeeding, *don't even think about taking any kind of illegal drug.* Period. And just to remind you about what's "illegal":

- *Marijuana.* The active ingredient in this drug is THC, which lingers in your baby's system for days and causes damage to the brain, plus affects DNA and RNA formation. Not to mention the fact that when you're stoned you're not exactly in the best frame of mind to parent a newborn.

- *Cocaine.* When you breastfeed your baby while using cocaine, your baby's health will take a turn for the worse: irritability, vomiting, dilated pupils, tremors, overstimulated heart and respiration are all possible, depending on the amount you take. By the way, cocaine stays in your milk for as long as sixty hours after exposure.

- *Heroin.* In addition to addicting your baby to heroin when you breastfeed on it, God knows what *else* is in that heroin, since it's rarely pure. And needless to say, when you're strung out on heroin, you're hardly an able parent.

A Word about Amphetamines

Technically, amphetamines are not illegal, but if you're abusing them, chances are you're obtaining them illegally and are taking far higher doses than was ever intended. Abuse of amphetamines can cause irritability and sleeplessness in the baby, because the drug is passed through breast milk.

If amphetamines are prescribed to you by a licensed doctor, ask whether you can still breastfeed. Take your doctor's advice, however, *not* your girlfriend's sister's. In certain circumstances, you can continue to breastfeed with a low dosage. If you're taking this medication for weight loss, you can stop; breastfeeding will do a better job.

Prescription Drugs

Okay, everybody, here are the official rules regarding prescription drugs and breastfeeding:

1. When a drug is prescribed, immediately inform your doctor that you're breastfeeding, and ask if the drug is safe *before* you fill the prescription.

2. If it isn't safe to use, explore whether alternative drugs can be substituted that are safe during breastfeeding. If not, you and your doctor will need to weigh the pros and cons of not taking the drug, delaying your therapy, early weaning, and so on. Just make sure you're making an informed decision.

3. If you're told that the drug is safe to use, and if the doctor who prescribed it is not your baby's doctor, then *before* you fill the prescription, consult your baby's physician too. If you're still given the green light, ask your pharmacist for a list of "contraindications" when you

fill the prescription. If breastfeeding is on that list, don't take the drug until you question your own doctor(s). And if it's not, keep in mind that much of the pharmaceutical literature is not useful when it comes to determining drug compatibility with breastfeeding. Review tables 2-1 to 2-5 on pages 46 to 55 for a list of drug interactions.

In general, two issues should always be addressed when questioning the safety of a prescription drug: How does the drug affect the baby? and How does the drug affect the ability to produce milk? Some drugs inhibit prolactin or oxytocin, affecting your milk supply and letdown, while others affect only the baby's health. In addition, the baby's age and weight contribute to your doctor's assessment of the safety issue. Finally, all doctors have several long lists of generic and brand-name drugs that affect breastfeeding. You can ask for copies of these lists to have on hand. See tables 2-1 and 2-2 for a list of the more common prescription and over-the-counter drugs that are unsafe (contraindicated) during breastfeeding.

Over-the-Counter Drugs and Herbs

The rules for over-the-counter drugs and herbs are a little trickier, since your doctor isn't with you in the pharmacy when you make your purchase. As for herbal remedies or beverages—be careful! Some of these are deadly. In this case, you need to work backward, and start by asking the pharmacist/herbalist the following questions:

1. Is breastfeeding contraindicated (unsafe) when taking this drug or herb?

2. What is the generic name of the drug or herb?

3. Are any side effects associated with this drug or herb?

4. Do any other medical conditions conflict with this drug or herb?

5. Do foods or other medications (such as prescription drugs) conflict with this drug or herb?

Then, *before* you take the drug or herb, consult your doctor and/or your baby's doctor about it too. Provide them with the following information by phone, fax, or e-mail:

- ๖ The brand name and generic drug or herb name
- ๖ Why you're taking it
- ๖ The dosage you plan to take
- ๖ How long you plan to take it

See tables 2-1 through 2-7 on pages 46 to 58 for a list of safe, less safe, and unsafe herbs.

Beware "Peer Information" about Drugs

When it comes to breastfeeding techniques and overcoming common problems, peer support groups and peer information is incredibly valuable. But . . . many women will call a peer or a peer-manned hotline about drugs and medications *instead* of a doctor or pharmacist. If you have a question about a drug, ask your doctor, not your friends! Medications are complicated, and a variety of factors may affect your doctor's decision to prescribe one over another.

WOMEN IN SPECIAL CIRCUMSTANCES

Because we live in an age where so many women are taking daily medications, managing chronic illnesses, or are cancer survivors, it's important to know whether you're a breastfeeding candidate or not.

Women Who May Not Be Able to Breastfeed

A number of rare conditions may actually make breastfeeding more harmful than formula. This is because breast milk is a *transmission route* for harmful viruses and medications. Alternatives to breastfeeding may be best, then, if you fall into any of the following categories:

♊ *Are on medications that are contraindicated during breastfeeding.* This includes chemotherapy drugs, as well as several other drugs used to manage long-term health problems.

♊ *Have an active infection or virus that can harm the baby.* Many exceptions apply, however. Women with hepatitis B, for example, can simply be immunized with the baby and then breastfeed as usual. Consult your doctor about your virus or infection (see pages 41 to 43).

♊ *Have silicone breast implants.* This is still in debate. See the section on implants on pages 38–40.

♊ *Do not have enough glandular tissue in your breast.* This is usually caused by breast surgery, discussed on page 37. In some cases, lactogogues may be supplied (more on this discussed in chapter 4).

If You Have Diabetes

So long as you're under the care of an endocrinologist and a primary-care physician or gynecologist, there's no reason why you can't breastfeed. In fact, breastfeeding reduces the need for insulin, so many diabetics find that their condition improves during lactation. This is particularly good news for women with gestational diabetes who may see their health bounce back that much quicker as a result.

If you are a candidate for a cesarean section (due to complications, common in diabetic births), it's important to arrange for help with breastfeeding prior to your scheduled delivery. Regardless of how you feed your baby, you should also discuss the possibility of insulin shock with your doctor prior to delivery, which is not uncommon due to fluctuating blood-sugar levels after delivery.

Common Obstacles to Breastfeeding

If you're insulin dependent, your insulin dosage may interfere with your prolactin levels at first, and this could delay your milk supply. Once your dosage is adjusted accordingly, your milk supply should establish itself. Until then, colostrum should be sufficient to nourish the baby, but stay in close touch with your baby's physician or nurse, who will note if the baby isn't thriving. An experienced nurse, midwife, lactation consultant, or La Leche League leader (see the appendix) will make sure that you're positioning the baby appropriately and will help you work toward encouraging your milk supply. Positioning may become of utmost importance to you especially, since diabetic women are prone to sorer nipples, thrush, and yeast infections in the nipples (discussed more fully in chapter 7).

Since many babies born to diabetic mothers have jaundice (50 percent of *all* babies have jaundice), colostrum is the best thing for them anyway. Colostrum will work as a laxative to help eliminate meconium from the intestines and prevent the absorption of bilirubin, the by-product that causes the jaundice. (Jaundice and bilirubin are discussed in detail in chapter 8.)

Diet

Whether your blood sugar is controlled by diet only or is helped with insulin, while breastfeeding you must stay under the strict supervision of a primary-care doctor, who may even refer you to a nutritionist and endocrinolgist. For one thing, you'll need to increase your calories without increasing your sugar or insulin dosage. And since milk production requires carbohydrates, you won't need as much insulin when you're nursing.

If your blood-sugar levels become too low, you'll develop hypoglycemia, which may cause the baby to lose weight (though you'd probably get the shakes and pass out before your baby's health would be affected). Regular glucose self-monitoring while under a doctor's care should ensure a good breastfeeding experience.

If You're Iron Deficient

It's common to become iron-deficient through blood loss from childbirth (just as it is through periods). But it's also important to note whether you're losing iron from other sources, such as blood loss in your stools. There's no reason not to breastfeed if you're iron-deficient. Iron, like calcium, can be ingested. The recommendation for women low in iron is to take an iron supplement: 200 mg/day of elemental iron, taken with vitamin C-containing foods (fruit, vegetables, and meat). Iron is much better absorbed with vitamin C and meat and is not absorbed as well in vegetarian diets. If your iron supplement upsets your stomach, liquid preparations are available, too.

Good sources of iron are organ meats (such as liver), poultry, fish, soybean, white beans, and lentils in combination with fruits and vegetables (or vitamin C). Tea and coffee can block iron absorption, so it's best to stay away or cut down.

If You're Expecting More Than One Baby

Breastfeeding is recommended for mothers of multiples. But you of all mothers-to-be should contact a lactation consultant before you deliver. Also, pick out a pediatrician prior to delivery. (Preparing for breastfeeding multiples is discussed in chapter 3.)

Women Who Work

Many women can comfortably manage breastfeeding despite a work schedule. In the past, women were encouraged to wean prior to returning to work, particularly if odd-hour shifts were involved. Today, with the aid of breast pumps and good information, working and breastfeeding is common. (Chapter 9 explores more fully how to balance a job and breastfeeding simultaneously.)

Women under Psychiatric Care

Unfortunately, if you're currently suffering from a biological depression of some sort, have bipolar disorder, or are receiving treatment for another condition, you are statistically at great risk for postpartum depression, which affects between 10 and 15 percent of the postpartum population. Even so, women can develop postpartum depression without having any history of a previous psychiatric illness.

This depression can begin at any time after delivery, from the first hours afterward to a few weeks later. The symptoms include decreased mood (apathy), loss of interest, change in appetite, fatigue, guilt, self-loathing, suicidal thoughts, and poor concentration and memory. When these feelings last for more than a couple of weeks, the consequences can be truly negative, leading to problems with bonding, breastfeeding, and relationships.

If you begin to notice these feelings, treatment is available with a qualified psychiatrist. You may just need some counseling, or you may need to be put on antidepressant medication. If you are taking medications for your condition, don't breastfeed before learning if your medications are breastfeeding-safe. Review table 2-3. The most recent studies show that breastfeeding is safe for women on amitriptyline, nortriptyline, desipramine, clomipramine, dothiepin, and sertraline. St. John's Wort, an herb, an effective, non-drug treatment for depression, is also safe to use while breastfeeding and may be worth trying before going on an antidepressant. Keep in mind, though, that sudden weaning can make depression worse and can even trigger depression.

When You've Had Breast Surgery

Whether you've had augmentation surgery, reduction surgery, cancer surgery, or reconstructive surgery, the answer to "Can I breastfeed?" greatly depends on whether any milk ducts or major nerves in the breast were cut or damaged. If they were not, then you should be able to breastfeed without difficulty.

If your incisions are located in the fold under your breast, chances are no milk ducts or nerves were damaged. If your incisions are near the armpits, then again, no damage was likely done. But if you have incisions around the areola or have had any breast tissue removed, then it's a safe bet that milk ducts were cut and that you may have some nerve damage too. Most breast-reduction surgery involves tissue removal, so your ability to produce milk will probably be reduced. In a 1990 study, researchers found that women with incisions around the areola were five times more likely to suffer from insufficient milk than women who had had more conservative incisions.

If you're unsure about what was and wasn't cut, contact your breast surgeon and find out. Then have a frank discussion with a lactation consultant about your breastfeeding chances.

In some cases, nipples are removed and reattached to make the breast more symmetrical. Nipples can also be burned either through injury or radiation therapy. When these things occur, breastfeeding is close to impossible, because the nipple either won't "work" or will be very sensitive, while scar tissue may prevent adequate milk letdown. Some women with bad burns have found, however, that the milk ducts reestablished, and they were able to breastfeed after all.

If you've had breast surgery that has damaged your milk ducts and nerves, or if your nipples have been burned, you may attempt breastfeeding as an experiment but be prepared to supplement if it doesn't work out. Also look into lactagogues, medications that trigger more milk.

If You Have Breast Implants

Breast implants are still a hotly debated topic among medical practitioners. To date, most lactation consultants will tell you that the feasibility of nursing with implants depends on the kind of implant you have, its age, and where it is placed.

Technically, if your implants are intact and were placed *behind* the milk ducts, milk production should not be affected. In some cases, however, the lobes and ductal system may have been disrupted by the implant surgery itself. Surgery may have also caused you to lose sensation in your breast if the nerve to the nipple and areola was severed. If there is nerve damage, it can interfere with your prolactin and oxytocin levels, which can totally disrupt your milk-ejection reflex and milk production.

But just because you *can* breastfeed with implants doesn't mean you should. Researchers are still concerned with two questions: First, if silicone breast implants do leak chemicals into the breast, do they get into breast milk and harm the suckling child? Second, if silicone implants cause some kind of immunological disease in the wearer, are there any biological consequences to a nursing child? Many women have gone on record to say that their children's health *deteriorated* after nursing with their implants in, while many childhood illnesses are blamed on "silicone milk" by an angry lay public.

There is some scientific evidence to back up these claims. A controversial 1994 study, published in the *Journal of the American Medical Association (JAMA)* concluded that babies who breastfed from mothers with silicone breast implants were at greater risk for "abnormal esophageal motility" (gastrointestinal problems). Symptoms would include abdominal pain, chronic vomiting, and poor weight gain. This study, however, has been widely criticized because it used a very small sampling of children, which critics argue makes the study irrelevant.

Another 1994 study questioned the relationship between silicone implants and autoimmune diseases in childhood, such as rheumatoid arthritis.

The American College of Allergy and Immunology, based in Illinois, announced in a 1993 press release that its findings clearly indicated that breast implants tend to ooze and rupture with age. When this happens, women are at risk for silicone-associated disorders, which cause chronic fatigue, pain, hair loss, and a variety of other symptoms. In their study, out of fifty-one women with breast implants who complained of muscle and joint aches and excessive fatigue, the breast implants had ruptured in over half of them, and all the women had had their breast implants in for at least ten years. Their research concluded that silicone in breast implants gradually oozes out to the outside surface of the implant, which can potentially get into the breast milk.

For what it's worth, in western Europe, women with silicone breast implants are advised against breastfeeding by the medical community because of the unknown health risks associated with them.

Are Your Implants Safe?
No one really knows. The dangers of silicone leakage are still being debated by an FDA advisory panel. Unfortunately, we still don't know how often silicone implants leak, how often they rupture, how long they last in the body, how much they leak, what happens to the body after a leakage, how often women with implants suffer adverse effects, or the best way to detect leaks and ruptures.

What we *do* know is that breastfeeding is dangerous if your breast implants have a polyurethane coating. Polyurethane releases TDA, a known carcinogen. However, these coatings have been banned for at least ten years.

What Should You Do?
If you feel uncomfortable with the lack of information regarding silicone implants and breastfeeding, you're not alone. The best advice is to follow that little voice inside you that says, "Hold on a minute!" In other words, if

you have implants, you may be better off not breastfeeding if you have any reservations about it. You don't want to put yourself in the position of constantly wondering about your child's health in years to come.

If You've Recently Found a Breast Lump

As soon as you discover a lump in your breast (before, during, or after pregnancy) see your doctor immediately to have the lump investigated. If you're already lactating, you most likely have a *milk cyst*, which is harmless and discussed in chapter 7. If you haven't yet delivered, a variety of things need to take place before you make your decision about breastfeeding:

1. Your lump needs to be aspirated by your doctor to see if it's a fluid-filled lump (a cyst), which is almost always benign.

2. If the lump is solid (i.e., not filled with fluid), you'll need a mammogram, and possibly a biopsy of the lump in a procedure known as a lumpectomy (where the lump is surgically removed). Most obstetricians will wait until you've delivered before carrying out these procedures, but it depends where you are in your pregnancy. A few weeks won't make a difference, but a few months may.

3. You will need to schedule a "Q & A" session with your breast-lump doctor to discuss how any of the planned procedures will affect breastfeeding. If a biopsy is unavoidable, and because of the location it is sure to damage some milk ducts and/or nerves, find out if it can be postponed to accommodate *some* breastfeeding time. (This, however, may not be practical.)

The Results

If your lump is benign, you can carry on with breastfeeding. Breast biopsies should not interfere with breastfeeding or weaning. Even if some milk ducts get cut, the rest of the breast will work fine. The areas that don't empty properly will get temporarily engorged (see chapters 4 and 7), but then will simply shut down, while the rest of the breast will just carry on.

If the biopsy results show cancer and further treatment is recommended, follow your doctor's advice. If you have to stop breastfeeding, don't feel guilty.

Breastfeeding and HIV/AIDS

If you're HIV-positive, meaning that your body has been exposed to the human immunodeficiency virus, the virus that causes AIDS, which stands for acquired immune deficiency syndrome, you should not breastfeed! It's been long established that HIV/AIDS can be transmitted from mother to child through breastfeeding. If you're not sure whether you are HIV-positive, it is your right to have confidential HIV testing. Discuss alternatives to breastfeeding with a lactation consultant or with your doctor.

A tragic case in point is the experience of the late AIDS activist Elizabeth Glaser (who died of AIDS), wife of actor Paul Michael Glaser. Elizabeth unwittingly passed on HIV to both her children when she breastfed; she had contracted the virus after receiving a blood transfusion in childbirth with her firstborn.

In 1996, 90 percent of all children who contracted HIV before age fifteen inherited the virus from their mothers during pregnancy, delivery, or breastfeeding, but recent data from developing countries indicates that up to one-half of mother-to-child HIV transmission is due to breastfeeding. Without treatment, the risk of HIV transmission between mother and child is greatest in poor countries (25 to 45 percent risk) or in poor parts of wealthy countries (15 to 25 percent risk in Europe or North America). Aside from pregnancy and breastfeeding, causes of high transmission rates in poor countries or areas are also due to a lack of access to drug treatment that can help prevent HIV transmission during pregnancy. Poor nutrition is also a factor. Some evidence suggests that women who are vitamin A deficient (vitamin A is abundant in leafy green vegetables and liver) are more likely to have HIV-positive babies. Research is now underway to determine whether vitamin A supplements in tablet form might reduce the risk of HIV-transmission in African women.

Formula in poor countries does not present a solution; it presents a dilemma. Health care workers must decide which risks are greater: the risk of the child contracting HIV through breast milk (25 to 40 percent risk), dying from infections against which breast milk offers protection, or dying from diarrhea as a result of ingesting infant formula made with contaminated water or animal milk when there is no access to safe water or refrigeration. There are also many areas where HIV testing is not available, or where formula is not affordable. Therefore, recommendations about breast-feeding to HIV-positive women in the Third World may vary.

In Thailand, where there is access to safe water HIV-positive women (they are tested at delivery) are cautioned against breastfeeding and encouraged to use formula, which is provided to them for free. Meanwhile, in sub-Saharan Africa, where childhood infections are common and HIV testing is often not available, breastfeeding is encouraged for all women. For example, if African mothers stopped breastfeeding, the death rate in children under five may double.

The Joint United Nations Programme on HIV/AIDS (known as UN-AIDS) now encourages countries to make HIV-positive mothers aware of the risks of breastfeeding versus formula feeding in their region so they can at least make an informed choice. It also encourages voluntary testing and counselling to be made more available.

The AZT Regimen

There is a way to prevent the transmission of HIV to your newborn if you are pregnant and HIV-positive and live in a developed country. In 1994, it was discovered that when the antiviral drug AZT was administered to HIV-positive women during pregnancy and to their newborns, the HIV transmission rate was reduced by 68 percent. Today HIV-infected women in the United States are routinely given AZT during the last twelve weeks of pregnancy, receive intravenous infusions of the drug during delivery, and then give the drug to their babies during their first six weeks of life. However, even if you live in an area where this drug is affordable, you should not breastfeed. There is still no clear evidence that suggests it is safe to breastfeed while receiving AZT; and nobody knows whether AZT is effective in preventing HIV transmission when the mother breastfeeds.

The effective AZT regimen (also known as the "076 regimen," after the number assigned to the federal study which proved it effective) costs roughly $1,000 (U.S.) per pregnant woman and newborn. Clearly, this is an expensive drug and unavailable in many places. In developing countries, where the government may have as little as $10 per person per year to spend on all health care, AZT is only available to the very wealthy or to women participating in clinical trials sponsored by agencies from industrialized countries. Even if AZT were affordable in all countries, prenatal care in general would need to be adequate enough for women to receive AZT in time. Right now, few women in developing countries have appropriate prenatal care and counseling about HIV. This reality led to one of the most explosive issues in medical ethics history: AZT trials in the Third World.

Officials at the United Nations, the World Health Organization, the National Institutes of Health in Bethesda, and the Centers of Disease Control in Atlanta wanted to find a way to develop a less expensive AZT regimen for pregnant HIV-positive women in poor countries. A "placebo study" seeks to establish whether the drug studied is actually better than nothing by giving a placebo to some study participants and the real drug to other participants. However, the guidelines for research ethics state that it is not ethical to withhold the best available treatment from a research subject. Withholding the AZT from some of the 12,211 study participants in Thailand, the Dominican Republic, Ethiopia, Ivory Coast, Uganda, Tanzania, and South Africa (where the trials took place) was criticized as unethical. In this trial, not only were human research subjects being denied the best available treatment, but babies born to women receiving a "dummy pill," or placebo, during the trial would be infected with HIV when researchers could have knowingly prevented it.

UNAIDS defended the trial arguing that the harsh reality in Africa is this: the Western AZT regimen is simply not available, and the only way to make any effective regimen available in poor countries is to test regimens against the current standard in those regions, which, in fact, is nothing. Furthermore, UNAIDS argued that all the women in the study were informed about the study's design and were aware that they may receive a placebo instead of a real drug.

The story ends with good news: U.S. government health officials announced in February 1998, that they are suspending placebo-controlled trials because a cheaper, and shorter regimen was found at $80 (instead of $1,000) per pregnant woman and newborn. The $80 regimen, given during the last four weeks of pregnancy, can cut transmission of HIV in half. (But $80 is still eight times what most developing nations spend per capita on health care each year.)

The success of the $80 treatment regimen depends on the fact that the women receiving the treatment do not breastfeed. So part of the "regimen" includes education on safe alternatives to breastfeeding. When there is no safe water or animal milk available, and no money to buy formula, how affordable is a breastfeeding alternative (not to mention the cost of HIV tests)? Efforts are therefore underway to bring down the costs in countries that cannot afford AZT, HIV testing, or formula.

ALTERNATIVES TO BREASTFEEDING

If you're unable to breastfeed or if it is medically inadvisable, please don't feel guilty. No one can do more than her best. Chapter 6 offers details about supplementing and feeding methods other than bottles.

Donor Milk

An excellent solution is to seek out donor breast milk from a friend, family member, or third person your doctor/midwife can recommend. If you're using donated breast milk from someone you know, make sure that she has been screened for HIV as well as the range of conditions that can affect breast milk, such as contraindicated medications and *risk* of HIV infection. You can discuss the appropriate "lab package" with your doctor, but the Red Cross screening guidelines used for donor sperm or eggs would be appropriate here.

Anonymous donor milk is also available. In fact, this is becoming such a popular solution, several "milk banks" are popping up all over North America. (See the appendix for a listing.)

Milk banks run on the same principle as sperm banks. All the milk donated is screened for harmful conditions, such as HIV, other viruses, or harmful medications. If you're using donor milk, HIV screening must be done. Thankfully, it's been found that by pasteurizing (a heat-treating process) human milk at 56 degrees Celsius for 30 minutes, *the HIV virus is killed!* Today, most milk banks make it standard practice to simply pasteurize (or "heat treat") all milk donations—regardless of HIV risk. *Make sure your milk bank does this.* If your donor milk is not going through a milk bank, call your local hospital and get instructions regarding heat treatment. At the proper temperatures with the proper equipment, it's possible to do this at home yourself. *Do not assume your donor is HIV-negative. Always heat treat donor milk!* If there are no milk banks in your area, however, and you cannot find a donor, you will have to use formula.

Formula

Ask your baby's physician to recommend a formula that is considered to offer the best nutrients. Obviously, the risks of formula—mainly the risk of serious illness (formula-fed babies get sicker and are hospitalized twice as often as breastfed babies)—must be balanced against the risks of potentially harmful breast milk. Because the risk of illness doubles when formula is used, breastfeeding advocates will call formula "harmful."

ℛ

For some of you, the information in this chapter may have indicated that you should not breastfeed. In this case, proceed to chapters 6, 8, and 10.

If you're all set for breastfeeding, the next chapter will give you the information you need to *prepare* for the event. Believe it or not, the prep work you do now will ensure far smoother sailing when that first feeding comes around. What if you can only partially breastfeed? Take a look at chapters 5 and 6, and then read chapter 3.

Table 2-1

DRUGS THAT ARE CONTRAINDICATED DURING BREASTFEEDING

Drug	Reason for Concern, Reported Sign or Symptom in Infant, or Effect on Lactation
Bromocriptine	Suppresses lactation; may be hazardous to the mother
Cocaine	Cocaine intoxication
Cyclophosphamide	Possible immune suppression; unknown effect on growth or association with carcinogenesis; neutropenia
Cyclosporine	Possible immune suppression; unknown effect on growth or assocation with carcinogenesis
Doxorubicin*	Possible immune suppression; unknown effect on growth or association with carcinogenesis
Ergotamine	Vomiting, diarrhea, convulsions (doses used in migraine medications)
Lithium	One-third to one-half therapeutic blood concentration in infants
Methotrexate	Possible immune suppression; unknown effect on growth or association with carcinogenesis; neutropenia
Phencyclidine (PCP)	Potent hallucinogen
Phenindione	Anticoagulant: increased prothrombin and partial thromboplastin time in one infant; not used in United States

*Drug is concentrated in human milk.

Reproduced by Permission of PEDIATRICS, *Vol. 93, copyright 1994.*

Table 2-2

Drugs of Abuse: Contraindicated during Breastfeeding*

Drug	Reported Effect or Reasons for Concern
Amphetamine†	Irritability, poor sleeping pattern
Cocaine	Cocaine intoxication
Heroin	Tremors, restlessnesss, vomiting, poor feeding
Marijuana	Only one report in literature; no effect mentioned
Nicotine (smoking)	Shock, vomiting, diarrhea, rapid heart rate, restlessness; decreased milk production
Phencyclidine	Potent hallucinogen

* The Committee on Drugs strongly believes that nursing mothers should not ingest any compounds listed in table 2-2. Not only are they hazardous to the nursing infant, but they are detrimental to the physical and emotional health of the mother. This list is obviously not complete; no drug of abuse should be ingested by nursing mothers even though adverse reports are not in the literature.

† Drug is concentrated in human milk.

Reproduced by Permission of PEDIATRICS, *Vol. 93, copyright 1994.*

Table 2-3

DRUGS WHOSE EFFECT ON NURSING INFANTS IS UNKNOWN BUT MAY BE OF CONCERN

Psychotropic drugs, the compounds listed under antianxiety, antidepressant, and antipsychotic categories, are of special concern when given to nursing mothers for long periods. Although there are no case reports of adverse effects in breastfeeding infants, these drugs do appear in human milk and thus could conceivably alter short-term and long-term central-nervous-system function.

Drug	Reported or Possible Effect
Antianxiety	
Diazepam	None
Lorazepam	None
Midazolam	. . .
Perphenazine	None
Prazepam*	None
Quazepam	None
Temazepam	. . .
Antidepressant	
Amitriptyline	None
Amoxapine	None
Desipramine	None
Dothiepin	None
Doxepin	None
Fluoxetine	. . .
Fluvoxamine	. . .
Imipramine	None
Trazodone	None
Antipsychotic	
Chlorpromazine	Galactorrhea in adult; drowsiness and lethargy in infant
Chlorprothixene	None
Haloperidol	None
Mesoridazine	None
Chloramphenicol	Possible idiosyncratic bone marrow suppression
Metroclopramide*	None described; dopaminergic blocking agent
Metronidazole	In vitro mutagen; may discontinue breastfeeding 12–24 hours to allow excretion of dose when single-dose therapy given to mother
Tinidazole	See metronidazole

*Drug is concentrated in human milk.

Reproduced by Permission of PEDIATRICS, *Vol. 93, copyright 1994.*

Table 2-4

DRUGS THAT HAVE BEEN ASSOCIATED WITH SIGNIFICANT EFFECTS ON SOME NURSING INFANTS AND SHOULD BE GIVEN TO NURSING MOTHERS WITH CAUTION*

Drug	Reported Effect
5-Aminosalicylic acid	Diarrhea (1 case)
Aspirin (salicylates)	Metabolic acidosis (1 case)
Clemastine	Drowsiness, irritability, refusal to feed, high-pitched cry, neck stiffness (1 case)
Phenobarbital	Sedation; infantile spasms after weaning from milk containing phenobarbital, methemoglobinemia (1 case)
Primidone	Sedation, feeding problems
Sulfasalazine (salicylazosulfapyridine)	Bloody diarrhea (1 case)

*Measure blood concentration in the infant when possible.

Reproduced by Permission of PEDIATRICS, *Vol. 93, copyright 1994.*

Table 2-5
MATERNAL MEDICATION USUALLY COMPATIBLE WITH BREASTFEEDING*

Drug	Reported Sign or Symptom in Infant on Lactation
Acebutolol	None
Acetaminophen	None
Acetazolamide	None
Acitretin	. . .
Acylovir[†]	None
Alcohol (ethanol)	With large amounts, drowsiness, diaphoresis, deep sleep, weakness, decrease in linear growth, abnormal weight gain; maternal ingestion of 1 g/kg daily decreases milk ejection reflex
Allopurinol	. . .
Amoxicillin	None
Antimony	. . .
Atenolol	None
Atropine	None
Azapropazone (apazone)	. . .
Aztreonam	None
B$_1$ (thiamin)	None
B$_6$ (pyridoxine)	None
B$_{12}$	None
Baclofen	None
Barbiturate	See table 2-4
Bendroflumethiazide (dicumarol)	Suppresses lactation
Bishydroxycoumarin (dicumarol)	None
Bromide	Rash, weakness, absence of cry with maternal intake of 5.4 g/day
Butorphanol	None
Caffeine	Irritability, poor sleeping pattern, excreted slowly; no effect with usual amount of caffeine beverages
Captopril	None

Table 2-5 continued

Drug	Reported Sign or Symptom in Infant on Lactation
Carbamazepine	None
Carbimazole	Goiter
Cascara	None
Cefadroxil	None
Cefazolin	None
Cefatoaxime	None
Cefoxitin	None
Cefprozil	. . .
Ceftazidime	None
Ceftriaxone	None
Chloral hydrate	Sleepiness
Chloroform	None
Chloroquine	None
Chlorothalidone	Excreted slowly
Chlorothiazide	None
Cimetidine[†]	None
Cisapride	None
Cisplatin	Not found in milk
Clindamycin	None
Clogestone	None
Clomipramine	. . .
Codeine	None
Colchicine	. . .
Contraceptive pill with estrogen/progesterone	Rare breast enlargement; decrease in milk production and protein content (not confirmed in several studies)
Cycloserine	None
D (vitamin)	None; follow up infant's serum calcium level if mother receives pharmacological doses
Danthron	Increased bowel activity

Table 2-5 continued

Drug	Reported Sign or Symptom in Infant on Lactation
Dapsone	None; sulfonamide detected in infant's urine
Dexbrompheniramine maleate with *d*-isoephedrine	Crying, poor sleeping patterns, irritability
Digoxin	None
Dilitazem	None
Dipyrone	None
Disopyramide	None
Domperidone	None
Dyphylline[†]	None
Enalapril	. . .
Erythromycin[†]	None
Estradiol	Withdrawal, vaginal bleeding
Ethambutol	None
Ethanol (cf. alcohol)	. . .
Ethosuximide	None, drug appears in infant serum
Fentanyl	. . .
Flecainide	. . .
Flufenamic acid	None
Fluorescein	. . .
Folic acid	None
Gold salts	None
Halothane	None
Hydralazine	None
Hydrochlorothiazide	. . .
Hydroxychloroquine[†]	None
Ibuprofen	None
Indomethacin	Seizure (1 case)
Iodides	May affect thyroid activity; see miscellaneous iodine

Table 2-5 continued

Drug	Reported Sign or Symptom in Infant on Lactation
Iodine (providone-iodine/vaginal douche)	Elevated iodine levels in breast milk, odor of iodine on infant's skin
Iodine	Goiter; see miscellaneous iodine
Iopanoic acid	None; acetyl metabolite also secreted; hepatotoxic
Isoniazid	None
K₁ (vitamin)	None
Kanamycin	None
Ketorolac	. . .
Labetalol	None
Levonorgestrel	. . .
Lidocaine	None
Loperamide	. . .
Magnesium sulfate	None
Medroxyprogesterone	None
Mefenamic acid	None
Methadone	None if mother receiving ≤ 20 mg/24 hours
Methimazole (active metabolite of carimazole)	None
Methocarbamol	None
Methyldopa	None
Methyprylon	Drowsiness
Metoprolol†	None
Metrizamide	None
Mexiletine	None
Minoxidil	None
Morphine	None; infant may have significant blood concentration
Moxalactam	None
Nadolol†	None

Table 2-5 continued

Drug	Reported Sign or Symptom in Infant on Lactation
Nalidixic acid	Hemolysis in infant with glucose-6-phosphate dehydrogenase (G-6-PD) deficiency
Naproxen	. . .
Nefopam	None
Nifedipine	. . .
Nitrofurantoin	Hemolysis in infant with G-6-PD deficiency
Norethynodrel	None
Norsterioids	None
Noscapine	None
Oxprenolol	None
Phenylbutazone	None
Phenytoin	Methemoglobinemia (1 case)
Piroxicam	None
Prednisone	None
Procainamide	None
Progesterone	None
Propoxyphene	None
Propranolol	None
Propylthiouracil	None
Pseudoephedrine[†]	None
Pyridostigmine	None
Pyrimethamine	None
Quinidine	None
Quinine	None
Riboflavin	None
Rifampin	None
Scopolamine	. . .
Secobarbital	None

Table 2-5 continued

Drug	Reported Sign or Symptom in Infant on Lactation
Senna	None
Sotalol	. . .
Spironolactone	None
Streptomycin	None
Sulbactam	None
Sulfapyridine	Caution in infant with jaundice or G-6-PD deficiency, and ill, stressed, or premature infant; appears in infant's milk
Sulfisoxazole	Caution in infant with jaundice or G-6-PD deficiency, and ill, stressed, or premature infant; appears in infant's milk
Suprofen	None
Terbutaline	None
Tetracycline	None; negligible absorption by infant
Theophylline	Irritability
Thiopental	None
Thiouracil	None mentioned; drug not used in United States
Ticarcillin	None
Timolol	None
Tolbutamide	Possible jaundice
Tolmetin	None
Trimethoprim/sulfamethoxazole	None
Triprolidine	None
Valproic acid	None
Verapamil	None
Warfarin	None
Zolpidem	None

*Drugs listed have been reported in the literature as having the effects listed or no effect. The word *none* means that no observable change was seen in the nursing infant while the mother was ingesting the compound. It is emphasized that most of the literature citations concern single-case reports or small series of infants.
† Drug is concentrated in human milk.

Reproduced by Permission of PEDIATRICS, *Vol. 93, copyright 1994.*

Table 2-6

FOOD AND ENVIRONMENTAL AGENTS: EFFECT ON BREASTFEEDING

Agent	Reported Sign or Symptom in Infant or Effect on Lactation
Aflatoxin	None
Aspartame	Caution if mother or infant has phenylketonuria
Bromide (photographic lab)	Potential absorption and bromide transfer into milk; see table 2-5
Cadmium	None reported
Chlordane	None reported
Chocolate (theobromine)	Irritability or increased bowel activity if excess amounts (16 oz/day) consumed by mother
DDT, benzenehexachlorides, dieldrin, aldrin, hepatachlorepoxide	None
Fava beans	Hemolysis in patient with glucose-6-phosphate dehydrogenase (G-6-PD) deficiency
Fluorides	None
Hexachlorobenzene	Skin rash, diarrhea, vomiting, dark urine, neurotoxicity, death
Hexachlorophene	None; possible contamination of milk from nipple washing
Lead	Possible neurotoxicity
Methyl mercury, mercury	May affect neurodevelopment
Monosodium glutamate	None
Polychlorinated biphenyls and polybrominated biphenyls facies	Lack of endurance, hypotonia, sullen expressionless
Tetrachlorethylene-cleaning fluid (perchloroehylene)	Obstructive jaundice, dark urine
Vegetarian diet	Signs of B_{12} deficiency

Table 2-7

Herbs Considered Safe in Moderation

Note: This table contains many herbs used for flavor in cooking. The small amounts used to flavor foods are safe. Caution is required, however, when using the larger amounts found in herb teas and medicinal herbal preparations. There is almost no information about the medicinal use of these herbs when breastfeeding; safest would be to avoid them completely.

Herb	Comments
Caraway	Contains carvol and carvene, which relax digestive-tract muscles. Traditional lactagogue, but no evidence for effectiveness.
Catnip	Contains nepetalactone, a hallucinogen for cats and probably a sedative for people.
Chamomile	Avoid if mother or baby have ragweed allergy. Contains bisabolol and others, which relax digestive-tract muscles. Traditionally used to reduce milk production, but no evidence for this.
Chickweed	
Cocoa, hot chocolate	Contains caffeine (see table 2-5). May cause esophageal reflux and heartburn.
Cola (kola nut)	Contains caffeine, theobromine, kolanin; all are stimulants. Basis of cola drinks.
Coriander	
Cranberry juice	Avoid if mother or baby allergic to cranberries. Helps prevent and clear urinary tract infections in mother.
Dill (leaf and seed)	
Garlic	Avoid if mother or baby allergic to garlic. Helps kill worms, bacteria, and fungi; prevents heart disease and stroke; helps eliminate lead from the body. Babies usually like the taste of garlic in breast milk.
Ginger root	Avoid in large doses. In China, used to induce menstruation at doses of 20–28 g, so large doses may cause miscarriage. Effective antinauseant. Ginger tea: 250 mg/cup; gingery food: 500 mg/serving; ginger ale: 100 mg/cup.
Kelp	Contains iodine and sodium alginate, which prevents heavy metal absorption. Effective for fibrocystic breast disease.
Kola nut (cola)	Contains caffeine, theobromine, kolanin; all are stimulants. Basis of cola drinks.
Lemon grass	
Marjoram	

Table 2-7 continued

Herb	Comments
Marshmallow	
Maté	Contains caffeine, tannins, vitamin C. Drink with milk to bind the tannins.
Mint leaves (spearmint, peppermint)	Avoid essential oils. Spearmint contains carvone, peppermint contains menthol; peppermint oil causes arrhythmias, and as little as a teaspoon of menthol can be fatal. Mints relax the gastroesophageal sphincter and can exacerbate reflux. Traditionally (England) used to reduce milk production.
Mullein leaf, flowers, roots	Avoid the seeds; mullein seeds are toxic. Contains mucilage, tannins.
Papaya leaf	Avoid if mother or baby are allergic to papaya.
Peppermint	Avoid the essential oil. Peppermint contians menthol; peppermint oil causes arrhythmias, and as little as a teaspoon of menthol can be fatal. Mints relax the gastroesophageal sphincter and can exacerbate reflux. Traditionally (England) used to reduce milk production.
Psyllium (Metamucil, etc.)	Avoid if mother or baby allergic to psyllium.
Raspberry leaf	Contains a uterine relaxant and tannins.
Rose hip	Contains vitamin C.
Rosemary	Contains antioxidant and antispasmodic.
Savory	Soothes the digestive tract; contains cineole, an expectorant.
Slippery elm	Avoid if mother or baby allergic to slippery elm. Contains mucilage.
Spearmint	Avoid essential oil. Contains carvone. Mints relax the gastroesophageal sphincter and can exacerbate reflux. Traditionally (England) used to reduce milk production.
Tea	Contains caffeine, theobromine, theophylline, tannins, fluoride. Take with milk to bind the tannins.

Compiled by Gillian Arsenault, M.D. from the following sources:
1. Castelman, M., and S. S. Hendler. *The Healing Herbs.* Rodale Press, Emmaus Pennsylvania, 1991: 36–380.
2. Hendler, S. S. *The Doctor's Vitamin and Mineral Encyclopedia.* Simon and Schuster, New York, 1990: 273–332.
3. Lawrence, R. A. *Breastfeeding: A Guide for the Medical Profession.* C.V. Mosby Co., St. Louis, 1989: 273–276.
4. Shrivastay, P., et al. Suppression of puerperal lactation using jasmine flowers (Jasminum sambac). Aust n Z J Obs Gynae 1988; 28:68–71.
5. Talalaj, S., and A. Czechowicz. Are Herbal Remedies Safe? (letter). Med J Aust, Jan 1988; 148:102–103.
6. ———. Cautions in the Use of Herbal Remedies during Pregnancy and for Small Children (letter). Med J Aust, Jan 1990; 152:52.

Table 2-8

HERBS TO USE WITH CAUTION

Note: This table contains many herbs used for flavor in cooking. The small amounts used to flavor foods are safe. Caution is required, however, when using the larger amounts found in herb teas and medicinal herbal preparations. There is almost no information about the medicinal use of these herbs when breastfeeding; safest would be to avoid them completely.

Herb	Comments
Alfalfa leaf	Contains saponins, which can destroy red blood cells.
Angelica (dong quai)	Contains psoralens (rash with sun exposure), and a laxative.
Anise	Contains plant estrogens (dianethole and photoanethole), which may suppress milk production.
Astragalus	Contains a diuretic that may suppress milk production. Used in cancer treatment in China.
Balm	Contains eugenol, which in excess causes nausea, vomiting, convulsions. May suppress thyroid function.
Barberry (see also goldenseal)	Contains berberine; in excess may cause nausea, vomiting, convulsions, hypotension, bradycardia, hypoventilation.
Basil	Contains estragol, which causes liver tumors in mice.
Bayberry	Contains myritictrin, gallic acid, tannins. Should be taken with milk to bind the tannins. In large doses, causes nausea, vomiting, sodium and potassium imbalance.
Bay leaf oil	Causes stupor and mild hypotension in animals.
Blackberry leaves, root, bark	Contains tannins. Should be taken with milk to bind the tannins. In large doses causes nausea, vomiting.
Black cohosh	Contains large amounts of plant estrogens, which may suppress milk production. In excess, may cause dizziness, nausea, vomiting, diarrhea, abdominal pain, dim vision, headache, shakiness, joint pain, bradycardia, and estrogenic side effects such as thrombosis and migraine.
Black haw	Contains scopoletin, used for menstrual cramps. Contains salicin, which can cause Reye's syndrome in children, and in excess can cause gastritis, nausea, vomiting, ringing in the ears.
Blessed thistle	Causes vomiting.
Borage leaf	Contains tannin, mineral acids.
Buchu	Contains a diuretic, which causes potassium loss and may reduce milk production.

Table 2-8 continued

Herb	Comments
Burdock (lappa, gogo)	Contains polyacetylenes and arctigenin. Contains a diuretic, which may reduce milk production. One report of atropine poisoning (blurry vision, dry mouth, hallucinations) from a burdock preparation, but may have been contaminated by belladonna.
Butcher's broom	Contains a diuretic, which may reduce milk production. May cause high blood pressure or bleeding problems.
Cascara	Contains anthraquinones, which are powerful laxatives. Contains aloe-emodin, which is toxic.
Celery seed	Contains a diuretic, which may reduce milk production. Contains phthalides (a sedative) and psoralins (rash with sun exposure).
Chaparral	Contains nordihydroguaiaretic acid (NDGA); in large doses may cause kidney and lymphatic disease in animals.
Cinnamon	Contains eugenol; in large doses causes nausea, vomiting, convulsions.
Clove	Contains eugenol; in large doses causes nausea, vomiting, convulsions.
Clover, red	Contains a plant estrogen, which may reduce milk production. Contains daidzein, genistein.
Dandelion	Contains a diuretic, which may reduce milk production. Contains a laxative.
Dong quai (angelica)	Contains a laxative. Contains psoralins (rash with sun exposure).
Echinacea	Contains echinacein. Not much information on use in children; no reports of toxicity in references used.
Elecampane	Contains alantolactone; expels worms and reduces blood pressure in animals. Sedative.
Ephedra (ma huang)	Contains ephedrine, a decongestant. Safer to use pseudophedrine (Sudafed, etc.).
Eucalyptus oil	Contains eucalyptol, which loosens phlegm, is antibacterial, and repels cockroaches, but is highly toxic. As little as one teaspoon has caused death. Dose is a maximum of 1–2 drops per cup of water.
Fennel seed	Contains anisic acid, a diuretic, which may reduce milk production. Has an estrogenic action, which may reduce milk production.
Fenugreek	Contains diosgenin, which acts like estrogen and may reduce milk production.
Feverfew	May cause bleeding problems. Good for migraine.
Gentian	Contains gentianine, which is anti-inflammatory and "stimulates stomach acid"; in excess may cause nausea, vomiting.
Ginko	Contains bioflavonoids, flavogylcosides, proanthrocyanides, polyacetones. May cause bleeding problems; in excess, may cause restlessness, nausea, vomiting.

Table 2-8 continued

Herb	Comments
Gogo (burdock, lappa)	Contains polyacetylenes and arctigenin. Contains a diuretic, which may reduce milk production. One report of atropine poisoning (blurry vision, dry mouth, hallucinations) from burdock preparation, but may have been contaminated by belladonna.
Goldenseal (similar to barberry)	Contains berberine; in excess causes nausea, vomiting, convulsion, hypotension, bradycardia, hypoventilation. Contains hydrastine, an antibiotic good for bacteria, fungi, and parasites; in large amounts, may cause death from cardia and respiratory arrest. Excess goldenseal can cause vomiting, leukopenia, and pins and needles in hands and feet. Sometimes an herb labeled "goldenseal" will actually be the cheaper bloodroot, which looks and tastes the same but is a powerful laxative and should *not* be taken when breastfeeding.
Gotu kola	Contains asiaticoside, which may cause cancer in animals. Large doses in animals have caused stupor and coma.
Hop	Contains plant estrogens, which may decrease milk production. Contains 2-methyl-3-butene-2-ol, a sedative.
Horehound	Contains marrubiin, an expectorant. In large amounts may cause arrhythmia.
Horsetail	Contains equisetonin (a diuretic), which may reduce milk production. Contains equisetine, a nerve poison (children using the stems as blowguns have been poisoned). Contains selenium, which may be present in toxic amounts, depending on soil grown in. Contains gold and thiaminase. Should be used for short periods if at all.
Hyssop officinalis	Contains marrubiin, an expectorant. Note: Do not take by mouth hedge hyssop (Gratiola officinalis); giant hyssop (Agastache); or water hyssop (Bacopa).
Jasmine	May reduce milk production.
Juniper (the flavoring in gin)	Avoid if allergic to juniper. Contains terpinen-4-ol, a diuretic, which may reduce milk production. In large doses, may cause kidney damage, hematuria, diarrhea, intestinal pain, tachycardia, hypertension.
Kavakava	Contains a diuretic, which may reduce milk production. Contains yangonin and pyrones, hallucinogens. One case of a man who drank 2 cups daily for 6 months, developing loss of balance, skin problems, and diarrhea; took one year to get better.
Lappa (burdock, gogo)	Contains polyacetylenes and arctigenin. Contains a diuretic, which may reduce milk production. One report of atropine poisoning (blurry vision, dry mouth, hallucinations) from a burdock preparation, but may have been contaminated by belladonna.
Licorice	Contains glyceyrrhetinic acid. Can cause hypertension, hypokalemia and hyonatremia, edema, diarrhea. In small amounts should be okay. One man who ate real licorice (most is artificially flavored these days) 2–4 oz/day for 7 years had to be hospitalized.

Table 2-8 continued

Herb	Comments
Lobelia	Contains lobeline, a euphoriant.
Ma huang (ephedra)	Contains ephedrine, a decongestant. Safer to use pseudophedrine (Sudafed, etc.).
Mandrake	Contains scopolamine and hyoscyamine.
Milk thistle	Contains silymarin and silybin.
Motherwort	Contains leonurine; may cause bleeding problems.
Myrrh	In large amounts, has a violent laxative effect.
Nettle	Contains a diuretic, which may reduce milk production. Traditional use as milk suppressant. Large doses of nettle tea can cause stomach irritation, burning skin, and trouble urinating.
Nutmeg	Contains myristicin, a hallucinogen.
Oregano	Contains carvacrol and thymol, expectorants.
Parsley	Contains apiol and myristcin, which are laxative and diuretic and may reduce milk production. Contains psoralens, which may cause rash with sun exposure.
Passion-flower (Passiflora incarnata)	Contains harmine alkaloids, which are sedative. Note: Do *not* take ornamental blue passion-flower (Passiflora caerula) by mouth; it contains cyanide.
Peppers, hot or red	Contain capsaicin. Some babies react when their mothers eat foods spiced with hot pepper. May cause bleeding problems in large amounts.
Periwinkle	Contains indole alkaloids, a hallucinogen.
Rhubarb stems	Contains anthraquinone laxatives. The leaves, which contain oxalic acid, are toxic and should not be eaten.
Saffron	Contains crocetin. In very large amounts, is toxic and has been fatal.
Sage	Can suppress breast-milk production. Contains tannins and an antiperspirant.
St. John's wort	Contains flavonoids and hypericin. Acts as a monoamine oxidase (MAO) inhibitor. Can increase sensitivity to the sun.
Sasparilla	Contains a diuretic and may reduce milk production. Large amounts can cause burning of mouth and throat and irritation of stomach and intestines.
Shepherd's purse	Causes blood clotting.
Skullcap	In large amounts, can cause confusion, twitching, and possibly convulsion.
Snakeroot (rauwolfia)	Contains reserpine, an antihypertensive.
Tarragon	Contains eugenol, which in large doses causes nausea, vomiting, and convulsions. Contains rutin. French tarragon is stronger than Russian tarragon.

Table 2-8 continued

Herb	Comments
Thorn apple	Contains atropine and scopolamine.
Thyme	Contains thymol and carvacrol. May cause a rash in sensitive people.
Turmeric	Contains curcumin; may reduce fertility; may cause bleeding problems.
Valerian	Contains valepotriates, which may reduce blood pressure. In large amounts, may cause headache, blurred vision, restlessness, nausea, morning grogginess. May interact with sedatives, hypnotics, antihistamines, analgesics.
Vervain	May cause bradycardia, bronchospasm, intestinal irritation, and uterine cramps.
Wild cherry	Contains hydrocyanic acid, which in large amounts can cause muscle spasms and twitching; has caused birth defects in animals.
Wormwood	Contains absinthin.
Yarrow	Avoid if allergic to ragweed (rash). Contains achielletin and achielleine, which cause blood clotting. Contains azulene, camphor, chamzulene, eugenol, menthol, quercetin, rutin, thuzone, and salicylates. In excess, can cause nausea, vomiting, and convulsions. May turn urine dark brown.
Yohimbe	Hallucinogen. May cause weight loss.

Compiled by Gillian Arsenault, M.D. from the following sources:
1. Castelman, M., and S. S. Hendler. *The Healing Herbs.* Rodale Press, Emmaus Pennsylvania, 1991: 36–380.
2. Hendler, S. S. *The Doctor's Vitamin and Mineral Encyclopedia.* Simon and Schuster, New York, 1990: 273–332.
3. Lawrence, R. A. *Breastfeeding: A Guide for the Medical Profession.* C.V. Mosby Co., St. Louis, 1989: 273–276.
4. Shrivastay, P., et al. Suppression of puerperal lactation using jasmine flowers (Jasminum sambac). Aust n Z J Obs Gynae 1988; 28:68–71.
5. Talalaj, S., and A. Czechowicz. Are Herbal Remedies Safe? (letter). Med J Aust, Jan 1988; 148:102-103.
6. ———. Cautions in the Use of Herbal Remedies during Pregnancy and for Small Children (letter). Med J Aust, Jan 1990; 152:52.

Table 2-9

HERBS TO AVOID COMPLETELY

Note: The following herbs can cause a variety of ill-health symptoms and/or severe reactions, some of which have been known to be fatal.

Herb	Comments
Alconite	Contains aconitine, a potent, fast-acting poison; causes respiratory and cardiac arrest.
Alfalfa seeds	Contains L-canavanine, which impairs red and white cell synthesis; may make SLE (lupus) worse.
Allspice oil	Contains eugenol; causes nausea, vomiting, convulsions.
Aloe vera	Fine for external use only. Do *not* apply to nipples when breastfeeding. Contains anthraquinones, which cause severe intestinal cramps and diarrhea. Contains salicylates (Reye's syndrome in children). May cause kidney inflammation.
Blue cohosh	Contains caulosaponin. Used to induce labor at term.
Boneset, dried	Contains pyrrolizidine alkaloids, which are hepatotoxic, and in large doses have been fatal.
Bonset, fresh	In addition to above, contains tremerol, which causes nausea, vomiting, weakness, tremor, hyperventilating, coma, and death.
Buckthorn	Contains a powerful laxative.
Cinnamon oil	Causes nausea, vomiting, and possible kidney damage.
Clover, sweet (melilot)	Contains natural coumarins, which impair clotting.
Coltsfoot (banned in Canada)	Contains pyrrolizidine alkaloids, which are hepatotoxic, and in large doses have been fatal.
Comfrey (banned in Canada)	Contains pyrrolizidine alkaloids, which are hepatotoxic, and in large doses have been fatal.
Crotolaria family	Contains pyrrolizidine alkaloids, which are hepatotoxic, and in large doses have been fatal.
Echium family	Contains pyrrolizidine alkaloids, which are hepatotoxic, and in large doses have been fatal.
Euphorbia resinifera	Powerful laxative. Causes vomiting.
Fennel oil	Causes trouble breathing, pulmonary edema, convulsions, and hallucinations.
Foxglove	Contains digitalis.

Table 2-9 continued

Herb	Comments
Ginseng	May cause insomnia, sore breasts, allergy symptoms, hypertension, arrhythmias, and masculining effects in women and feminizing effects in men. (Asian tradition is to use in the elderly; not in children.)
Golden wort	Contains pyrrolizidine alkaloids, which are hepatotoxic, and in large doses have been fatal.
Hawthorn	Contains cardioglycosides; heart stimulants and hypotensives.
Helitropium family	Contains pyrrolizidine alkaloids, which are hepatotoxic, and in large doses have been fatal.
Hound tongue	Contains pyrrolizidine alkaloids, which are hepatotoxic, and in large doses have been fatal.
Mandrake	Contains podophyllin.
Meadowsweet	Contains salicylates (Reye's syndrome in children).
Melilot (sweet clover)	Contains coumarins, which inhibit coagulation.
Mistletoe	Contains tyramine; may cause fatal hypertension in those taking MAO inhibitors; children have died from as few as 2 mistletoe berries.
Necio family	Contains pyrrolizidine alkaloids, which are hepatotoxic, and in large doses have been fatal.
Pennyroyal leaves	Contains pulegone.
Pennyroyal oil	Highly toxic; one case of death 2 hours after taking 2 tablespoons of the oil.
Pokeroot	Contains phytolaccatoxin, which is highly toxic; may cause leukopenia even when used externally.
Ragwort	Contains pyrrolizidine alkaloids, which are hepatotoxic, and in large doses have been fatal.
Rosemary oil	Even small amounts can cause stomach, kidney, and intestinal poisoning.
Sassafrass	Contains safrole, which may cause cancer.
Savine	
Senna	A powerful laxative.
Sweet flag	Contains beta-asarone, which causes cancer in animals.
Tansy	
Tea tree oil	Do not put on nipples when breastfeeding.

Table 2-9 continued

Herb	Comments
Thyme oil	Even a few teaspoons can cause headache, nausea, vomiting, thyroid problems, bradycardia, and hypoventilation.
Tonka beans	Contains natural coumarins, which inhibit coagulation.Uva Ursi Contains a diuretic, which may reduce milk production. Contains arbutin, which breaks down to hydro-quinone; in large doses may cause vomiting, tinnitus, and delirum. Contains tannins (take with milk). May turn urine green. May be hepatotoxic in children.
White willow	Contains salicytates (Reye's syndrome in children).
Witch hazel	May be used as an external compress or gargle, but do not take internally or apply to nipples when breastfeeding.
Woodruff	Contains natural coumarins, which inhibit coagulation.

Compiled by Gillian Arsenault, M.D. from the following sources:
1. Castelman, M., and S. S. Hendler. *The Healing Herbs*. Rodale Press, Emmaus Pennsylvania, 1991: 36–380.
2. Elliot, C. Tea tree oil poisoning. Med J Australia; 1993, 159(6): 830–831.2.
3. Hendler, S. S. *The Doctor's Vitamin and Mineral Encyclopedia*. Simon and Schuster, New York, 1990: 273–332.
4. Lawrence, R. A. *Breastfeeding: A Guide for the Medical Profession*. C.V. Mosby Co., St. Louis, 1989: 273–276.
5. Seawright, A. Tea tree oil: comment. Med J Australia, 1993; 159(6):831.
6. Shrivastay, P., et al. Suppression of puerperal lactation using jasmine flowers (Jasminum sambac). Aust n Z J Obs Gynae 1988; 28:68–71.
7. Talalaj, S., and A. Czechowicz. Are Herbal Remedies Safe? (letter). Med J Australia, Jan 1988; 148:102–103.
8. ———. Cautions in the Use of Herbal Remedies during Pregnancy and for Small Children (letter). Med J Australia, Jan 1990; 152:52.

chapter 3

PREPARING FOR BREASTFEEDING

Your reading this book is itself a large part of preparing for breast-feeding. Learning about the process and the physiology involved with lactation makes a huge difference in your breastfeeding experience. In other words, you're not just learning to drive, but about how the car *works*—an important step in preparing for any journey. But like any road trip, the difference between a smooth ride and a rough one on the breastfeeding highway is largely knowing what to pack, and who to bring along! Consider this chapter breastfeeding triptych and camp list all in one. (By the way, to make this chapter as lean as possible, I've left out the details on baby furniture and rocking chairs.)

WHO IS YOUR BREASTFEEDING PRACTITIONER?

There are so many things to know about the breastfeeding process, it's amazing it hasn't become a specialty of its own in medicine, yielding a host of able "lactologists." Although such a practitioner would be wonderful to turn to, in the real world that person doesn't exist. As a result, breastfeeding women today need to establish a team of practitioners they can turn to for information, lactation help, and general troubleshooting: a lactation consultant (discussed next); a good general or family doctor for your baby (or, as is common in large urban areas, a pediatrician); and your own primary-care physician (who may also be your baby's doctor). Have the names and phone numbers of this trio prior to delivery to ensure the best possible care for you and the baby. If a problem arises soon after birth, for example, you may want immediate access to one of these practitioners. There may not be a lot of time to spare.

In Search of a Lactation Consultant

A lactation consultant (LC) is the equivalent of a breastfeeding "midwife." These women are trained to help new mothers learn the technique of breastfeeding; provide information about breastfeeding; and solve problems that arise during breastfeeding. They offer guidance on anything from positioning and latch difficulties to nutrition, first baby solids, and even contraception.

Many certified lactation consultants are nurses and/or certified nurse-midwives who have obtained their LC status by taking postgraduate-degree courses and a written exam. When they pass the exam, they earn the initials "I.B.C.L.C.," which stand for International Board Certified Lactation Consultant. This degree must be renewed every five years thereafter. In some cases, LCs have a masters of science degree without a nursing degree, but a number of primary-care doctors and some specialists are now matriculating to become LCs too. You can find out if a lactation consultant is board certified by calling (703) 560-7330.

It's best to get the name of a lactation consultant prior to delivery. If breastfeeding goes well, you probably won't need to see one, but if breastfeeding presents problems for you, the consultation may save your breastfeeding experience. Sometimes you needn't go farther than your own nurse-midwife, who will simply continue to see you through lactation.

The first place to start looking for an LC is your pregnancy practitioner. Whether you're under the care of an obstetrician, a primary-care physician, or a midwife, ask to be referred to an LC sometime in the third trimester. Many doctors and midwives have lists of LCs on hand, but don't be surprised if you're asked, "What's an LC?"

Your hospital or birthing facility may have an LC on staff. Many do, some don't. If all else fails, refer to the appendix for a list of organizations that can give you names of good LCs.

Who Should Consult an LC?

It is especially crucial to find an LC if you're carrying multiple fetuses, since your gestation period may be shorter than that of a woman carrying a single baby.

First-time breastfeeders who do not anticipate any problems should be able to gather sufficient information by attending a La Leche League meeting, for example. But even if this is your second or third child, keep in mind that every child *feeds* differently, and may present unique challenges you're not prepared for.

Anyone anticipating problems with breastfeeding after delivery should absolutely consult an LC. This includes:

- some mothers with inverted or flat nipples who cannot fix the problem themselves
- mothers whose breasts have not enlarged during pregnancy
- mothers of multiples
- mothers of children with certain disabilities (you know who you are)
- mothers who are experiencing a high-risk pregnancy (you know who you are)
- mothers who have had breast surgery (biopsies not included)
- mothers managing other chronic health conditions

When to Consult an LC

Your seventh or eighth month of pregnancy is usually the best time to have your first visit with an LC. Most women deliver anywhere from two weeks before to two weeks after their due date, so don't leave it to the last minute.

The first visit is designed to get you acquainted with your LC and give you a chance to ask questions about breastfeeding, get her business card so you can call her when you deliver, verify her credentials, and even explore her breastfeeding philosophy to see if you're compatible. Let her know, too, where you're giving birth, so she can visit you in the first few hours after delivery.

Seeing an LC prior to the birth will also facilitate a calmer first meeting, when you're less anxious and less overwhelmed.

The Costs

LCs are not free. As with any consultant, most LCs charge by the hour. Rates vary from state to state (or province to province), but the average home visit costs about $40. Your hospital's LC will not charge for the time she spends with you in the hospital, but she will if she sees you elsewhere. To date, virtually no health-care plan covers the cost of an LC.

Meet Your Baby's Doctor

Whether you're having one child or are anticipating twins or a child with mental or physical disabilities, you will need to provide that child with a good general or family practitioner. In large cities, pediatricians, whose practices were once confined to more seriously ill or exceptional children, now handle general-practice concerns as well and are often considered primary-care doctors for children.

If your pregnancy is being managed by an obstetrician or primary-care physician, both these doctors will have lists of children's doctors they can refer you to. The best time to seek out one is in the third trimester, so you can take your time in choosing one who best meets with your own philosophies of child rearing and breastfeeding.

For example, despite all the research in the medical literature, many children's doctors still don't support breastfeeding at all and feel that formula is fine. Others support breastfeeding to a point. One woman's pediatrician recommended formula after only four weeks of nursing, telling her, "Once you've given the baby your colostrum, there's no real point in continuing unless you want to." This mother began giving the child formula and, sure enough, stopped producing enough milk for a full-time milk supply.

Here are some questions you might want to consider before you sign on as a new patient:

1. *Do you like the way the business is set up?* Medical practices come in three basic setups: solo practices (just the doctor and a support staff); partnerships (two or more doctors sharing patients, costs, and space); or combination practices (a collection of different specialists

under one roof, who all work as a kind of team. There's no right or wrong setup, just what you're most comfortable with.

2. *How does the doctor feel about your decision to breastfeed?* Make sure the doctor supports your decision to breastfeed and is willing to work with you to solve breastfeeding problems—not just hand you a bottle when all may not be going well.

3. *Where is the doctor located?* Is the office close by, or does it take you over an hour to get to? Traipsing across town with a baby just to go to the doctor will add unnecessary stress to your life.

4. *Can you reach the doctor by phone?* Can you just pick up the phone and call when you're worried about your baby's health and don't know what to do? If you can't, is it because the doctor is truly busy or just not accessible? Doctors should leave an emergency number you can call after hours.

5. *If this weren't your child's doctor, would you want him or her as a friend?* If you wouldn't be caught dead having a cup of coffee with this doctor, why would you allow him or her access to your child?

6. *Does this doctor make house calls?* House calls in larger urban areas are beginning to come back into vogue in situations that warrant a home visit—definitely a bonus when you have a newborn.

7. *How long has this doctor been practicing?* Sometimes, the older the doctor, the less supportive he or she may be of breastfeeding in general. Younger doctors may be more open and up-to-date.

8. *Has this doctor ever breastfed?* If the doctor had a good breastfeeding experience herself, then she's likely to be truly supportive of the process and knowledgeble in problem solving—no matter how old she is. But if this doctor had a bad breastfeeding experience, she may be the worst choice of all, out to prove that no one can breastfeed any better or longer than she did.

9. *Who backs up the doctor?* Request to meet the "backup" doctor who fills in on weekends, off-hours, or when the regular doctor is on vacation—before you come aboard.

10. *Can the practice refer you to an LC if necessary?* If the doctor has a few names on hand, this is a good sign.

Red Flags

If you hear your doctor say any of the following statements, he or she obviously doesn't know much about breastfeeding:

- "Here are some free formula samples and company literature to take home."

- "Breastfeeding and formula are equivalent."

- "Brand X formula is best."

- "It's not necessary to feed your baby right after birth since you'll be tired, and/or the baby will not be hungry."

- "There's no such thing as nipple confusion."

- "If you or the baby is sick, you should stop breastfeeding."

- "I'm surprised that your six-month-old is still breastfeeding because there is no value in breast milk or breastfeeding beyond six months."

Other Questions to Ask

Once you've selected this doctor, you might ask the following questions at some point prior to delivery to help you prepare for situations where medical intervention may be necessary.

1. *What conditions do you feel warrant supplementing breast milk with sugar water or formula, and how do you advise giving supplements?* (If the doctor can't think of anything but a bottle, this physician's not up-to-date!)

2. *How can I tell if my baby is thriving? What warning signs should I watch for that would indicate a problem?*

3. *Given my own medical history, is there any particular problem I should anticipate with respect to my newborn's health or my ability to breastfeed?*

If You're Expecting Multiples

You'll most likely be dealing with a pediatrician in this case, who may be put in charge of your case upon delivery. It's a good idea to find out who this doctor is and make an appointment prior to the birth to discuss some of the standard care procedures of mulitiples.

You'll also find that many pediatricians are less supportive of breast-feeding if you're expecting multiples. Here are some questions to ask the pe-diatrician, which will help pinpoint differing philosophies from the outset:

1. *How much experience do you have with patients who have breastfed multiples?*

2. *Do you believe that multiples can be totally breastfed? For how long?*

3. *If one or more of my babies requires special care, I plan to express milk for them. Under what circumstances would my babies NOT be able to receive my milk?*

Women in Special Circumstances

If you fall into some of the special circumstances discussed in chapter 2 (see page 33), discuss your decision to breastfeed with your pregnancy practi-tioner, and possibly your baby's doctor, an LC, and/or the specialist who normally manages your condition. Whether you had breast surgery, have breast implants, or are an insulin-dependent diabetic, you'll need to find out how breastfeeding will affect your condition. You'll also need to get a list of warning signs that may signify that you're either not producing enough milk or that the baby isn't thriving.

What More Can You Do?

Once you've chosen a doctor for your baby and have the name of an LC (in case of problems) or have met with one because you're at risk for having problems, you may choose to prepare your breasts for breastfeeding. This can be done either by having your partner suck and caress your breasts during lovemaking (don't do this if you are threatening to deliver prematurely) or giving yourself a gentle breast massage. In addition, in the last few weeks of pregnancy, you may want to try to express some colostrum yourself (which may leak out anyway).

Now is also a good time to put breastfeeding on your birth plan, investigate breast pumps, and educate yourself about all the breastfeeding accessories you may or may not be needing.

IS BREASTFEEDING ON YOUR BIRTH PLAN?

For those of you who have read *The Pregnancy Sourcebook,* I describe the birth plan as a sort of labor-and-delivery "wish list" that helps you control as much of your delivery destiny as possible. While birth plans don't always go according to expectations, many women forget to include certain provisions that would ensure a better start to breastfeeding after the delivery is over. Here are some suggestions:

1. Make it known that you want to breastfeed. (Try to find a baby-friendly hospital.)

2. Demand rooming-in privileges. This means your baby sleeps in the room with you, and not in a standard nursery. That way, when it's time to feed you'll be there at the early stage of hunger, when the baby's most likely to latch on (as opposed to howling in frustration). Sharing close quarters will help to synchronize your respective sleep cycles; the baby will more likely rouse when it's easier for you to wake up—and then fall back asleep!

3. Leave some instructions for the neonatal nursing staff. You'll want to make sure that the nursing staff is not giving your newborn a bottle or a pacifier. Basically, artificial nipples encourage a tongue-thrust habit that leads to "nipple confusion." This will not only interfere with suckling at your breast but will make hamburger out of your nipple. Make sure, too, that the nursing staff does not unnecessarily supplement your newborn with sugar water. Many hospitals now

give some dehydrated newborns a small quantity of sugar water via a cup or feeder, which may interfere with breastfeeding unless it's given by feeding tube at the breast (see chapter 6).

4. If possible, reserve time with a nurse, midwife, or LC for "getting started" lessons. If the hospital has an LC on staff, see if you can reserve some time with her the first or second day after birth so you can discuss any problems you may be having.

5. Ask to hold the infant (if healthy) right after birth. This is when you're euphoric and the baby is quietly alert and searching. It's also the best time for you and Dad to hold the baby, cuddle, and talk to each other, and for the baby to nuzzle and begin to lick your nipple. If you can't hold the baby right away, then just do it as soon as the baby's health signs indicate you can. Even if you have had a cesarean delivery, the ASAP rule can still be followed.

6. Request a list of all tests, medications, and/or supplements given to your newborn in your absence.

Provisions for Multiples and/or Premies

Since multiple pregnancies tend to have a shorter gestation period (the more babies, the more likely you are of delivering earlier), the result may be premature babies. In this case, breastfeeding is actually *more* crucial, but sometimes less supported. For single births that are premature, breastfeeding is also a crucial element in the infant's survival.

If your baby(ies) is/are staying in a neonatal care unit, state on your birth plan that you want these babies fed colostrum *only*, which you can express yourself with a pump. (Pumps are discussed further below; expression is discussed in detail in chapter 5.)

If you're expecting to deliver prematurely, you can arrange on your birth plan to have a full-size automatic electric breast pump made available to you at the hospital in case you're separated from one or more of your babies after birth.

With respect to multiples, the obvious question that needs to be addressed is Will you have enough milk? The answer is yes. Remember, your breasts work on sheer demand and supply. The more, the merrier; the more suckling, the more milk production. The problem with feeding two or more mouths is that you may never get *relief* from feeding, unless you design a schedule that's workable. In addition, because your positioning is trickier to coordinate, you of all mothers will benefit from meeting with a lactation consultant as well as a visit from that LC within the first two days of delivery.

In order to plan for breastfeeding more than one baby, you *must* arrange for help at home. Attend to these arrangements prior to delivery. You need not look into hiring a trained British nanny, but simply a good domestic housekeeper to help you with chores, not baby care. You and your LC can also work together to plan a workable feeding schedule. (See chapter 4 for more details.)

The Baby-Friendly Hospital Initiative

There is currently a worldwide effort, led by UNICEF and WHO (World Health Organization), to make hospitals "baby friendly," wherein they adopt practices that support breastfeeding. For example, the UNICEF executive board has called on governments in industrialized countries to end the distribution of free or low-cost formula. In order for a hospital to be classified as baby friendly (which may involve a future logo or seal on the hospital's doors), ten requirements developed by UNICEF and WHO must be met. These hospitals must:

1. Have a written breastfeeding policy.

2. Train all health staff to implement this policy.

3. Inform all pregnant women about the benefits of breastfeeding.

4. Help mothers initiate breastfeeding within half an hour of birth.

5. Show mothers the best way to breastfeed.

6. Give newborn infants no food or drink other than breast milk, unless medically indicated.

7. Practice rooming-in by allowing mothers and babies to remain together twenty-four hours a day.

8. Encourage breastfeeding on demand.

9. Give no artificial nipples.

10. Foster the establishment of breastfeeding support groups and refer mothers to them upon discharge from the hospital or clinic.

The questionnaire on pages 126 to 127 will help you decide how baby-friendly your own hospital is.

A CONSUMER'S GUIDE TO BREAST PUMPS

Key to good breastfeeding planning is looking into a breast pump *prior* to delivery in the event you have trouble getting started. A breast pump will ensure that your milk supply is kept up, even if breastfeeding isn't going that well at first. And, as discussed just above, if you're giving birth to multiples or deliver prematurely, you'll need a breast pump at your bedside in the hospital to express the milk that your babies will be fed in the neonatal unit.

You can express your milk by hand (directions provided in chapter 5), but hand expression takes some time to master. Good pumps empty the breast faster—some even work both breasts simultaneously. As in any consumer product, the adage buyer beware particularly applies here. So read on for what you need to know about breast pumps before you rent, lease, or buy.

Hand-Expression Funnel

If you want to try your hand at expressing, this is one product to use. The hand-expression funnel is made of hard, lightweight plastic. Sterilize the funnel and collection bottle before you first use it. After that, wash the funnel and the collection bottle in lukewarm, soapy water, rinse in clear water, and then air dry. This method operates on the principles of basic physics: The deep, cup-shaped opening of the hand-expression funnel is large enough to fit your hand and breast, while the rolled rim facing inward is designed to catch all the sprays of expressed milk. The funnel is sized to fit onto any standard feeding bottle. The advantage of hand-expression—if you're efficient at it—is that it's cheap, goes where you do, and doesn't require batteries or electricity. The downside is that it may take some time to work up the hand muscles necessary to do this efficiently.

Manual Pumps

Unlike electric pumps, manual pumps are quieter, smaller, easier to carry, and often easier to wash. You don't need to worry about batteries or plugging them in. Some manual pumps can be operated with one hand, which means that you can empty both breasts simultaneously if you have two pumps.

Best Pumps/Worst Pumps

The best of these are the cylinder-type pumps, which require two hands to operate, or the one-hand pumps.

In a cylinder-type pump, one cylinder fits inside another, with a rubber gasket acting as a seal between. Suction and pressure are created when the inner cylinder is pulled out, drawing the milk into the outer cylinder or a separate collection bottle. Most cylinder-type pumps are dishwasher safe (gaskets may need to be hand washed), and some models have adapters that can adjust shields to different breast sizes (the shields on some models are angled so that pumping is awkward or tiring). You can also use a cylinder pump if you're lying on your side.

Unless you have a model with a separate collection bottle, the pump can easily tip over and the milk can get inside the rubber gasket, which will interfere with the pumping action. With a collection bottle, you don't have to stop pumping to empty the pump, and the suction you generate is more level. Finally, you may need to frequently empty the pumped milk into another container as the milk level rises, which will interfere with the pumping.

Manual aspirator pumps are less effiecient. Here you actually suck on one of two tubes, which extends from the top of a collection bottle. This creates a vacuum in the bottle that provides the suction and pressure to stimulate the breast and draw the milk out from the breast into the other tube and the collection bottle. The advantage of this model is that you can pump while you're lying down, but the suction and pressure usually aren't strong enough to empty your breasts effectively.

Ye Olde Bicycle Horns

Don't go anywhere *near* the rubber bulb–type "bicycle horn" pumps (aka "nipple killers"). Not only do bicycle-horn pumps fail to empty your breasts, they can damage breast tissue because of poor pressure and also damage your nipples, causing sorness and redness. The way they work is that the rubber bulb is squeezed, causing suction, which provides pressure and draws the milk into the pump. The only advantages are they're cheap, small, and portable. But since they're hard to clean and can't be sterilized, the milk can easily be contaminated.

A supposedly "new and improved" version of the bicycle-horn pump does have a separate collection bottle for milk, can be sterilized, and offers "adjustable" suction (on models that have a suction moderator). But even these models can pinch your nipples and cause soreness. Stay away.

Trigger-Happy

Trigger-action pumps are another manual pump product. Here you pull a trigger like one on a Windex bottle to generate the suction and pressure you need. Except in this case, imagine spraying onto yourself (holding the trigger backward). These do come with a separate collection bottle, but they're a little more expensive than other manually powered pumps, and they require more strength and energy to operate. (Not recommended for women with small hands!) A major downside to the trigger pump is that some models have a glass breast shield, which is breakable and expensive to replace. The advantage is that you can pump both breasts at once.

Electric Pumps

Electric pumps are bigger, heavier, harder to wash, and noisier, but the good ones can empty a breast much faster than manual pumps, while some have a double setup, which allows you to pump both breasts at the same time.

Best Pumps/Worst Pumps

The best kind of electric pump has an automatic cycle for the suction pressure, which imitates a baby's suckling cycle. You simply adjust the pressure-level control knob, sit back, and let the pump do the work.

Since these pumps are expensive, it's probably best to rent one. A good electric pump will run about three dollars a day (less than a day's worth of formula) to rent. If you need to pump several times a day, this is your best bet.

The only kind of electric pump to avoid is the kind that requires you to turn the suction on and off yourself (usually by sliding your thumb on and off a hole in the suction system).

You Can't Take It with You

The biggest disadvantage to an electric pump is that it's not very portable. When you have to go out or travel, use a manual cylinder or trigger-style pump or else just hand-express.

Batteries Not Included: Battery-Operated Pumps

Battery-powered motors cannot provide uninterrupted suction. So in order to use these, you need to interrupt the suction pattern by putting your finger over the suction-release valve or depressing a lever or button.

On the other hand, battery-operated pumps can be operated with one hand, giving you the option of pumping while the baby nurses on the other breast or double pumping by using two hand pumps simultaneously. They're also small and portable. Batteries need to be changed frequently, however, often every two to three days. When batteries are running low, the suction is poor, which does not allow the breast to empty effectively.

The AC/DC Pump

The AC/DC pump goes both ways; it can be powered by batteries or electricity. It works on a small, fish-tank-style motor, providing continuous suction and negative pressure, which you will need to interrupt to mimic a baby's sucking pattern. Users report that this pump works best if it's warmed up for a few minutes prior to use. The AC/DC pump has the same disadvantages of battery-powered pumps if you're using battery power. Otherwise, it can be used as an adequate electric pump, and is lightweight, portable, and easy to clean. The shield on some of the hand-held electric models is poorly designed, however, making it less effective. In addition, this type of pump tends to vibrate when resting on a flat surface, which can cause spills.

Other Products and Accessories

Once you've got your breast pump, there are some other things you might need, such as specially designed human milk bags (you can use existing kitchenware, too), information on storage, as well as alternative feeders in case you need to supplement. (All these products are discussed in chapter 5.)

BOOBY TRAPS

You may have been talked into purchasing a variety of products prior to delivery. Those discussed in this section range from ineffective to outright damaging. Here's the list of breast products from hell that lactation experts suggest you avoid.

Breast Shells

I briefly discussed these in chapter 1. Also called milk cups, breast cups, breast shields, or Woolwich shields, breast shells are made of hard, lightweight plastic resembling an areola with a hole in the center for either a flat or inverted nipple to stick out of. These are not designed to be worn during breastfeeding, but prior to delivery or between feedings to "train" an inverted or flat nipple to come out. They don't work. To bring out an inverted or flat nipple, see Preparing Inverted or Flat Nipples on page 84.

Breast shells are designed to be worn inside your bra, but unless you wear a bra that is one cup size larger than usual to accommodate them comfortably, the pressure from the shells can cause mastitis, or inflammation of the breast, which we discuss further in chapter 7.

Moreover, unless the shells are washed daily and sterilized weekly, bacteria tend to get inside the breast via the Montgomery glands (see chapter 1), which can cause a range of nasty infections.

Breast shells become dangerous once you begin feeding because they don't allow adequate drying of the nipples between feedings, which can cause nipple soreness and more mastitis. What's worse, some women leak milk into the breast shell while it is worn. This milk stays warm and close to the body, grows bacteria, and causes even more nasty infections.

The Kiss of Death: Nipple Shields

Nipple shields are soft latex, silicone, or rubber nipples that are designed to be worn *over* your nipples during feedings. These things, which destroy your milk supply, were invented to help women with sore nipples continue nursing. Sore nipples are caused by a poor latch. In order to become *un*sore, *the latch problem needs to be corrected first.* (See chapter 7 for more information on treating sore nipples; see chapter 4 for information on establishing a good latch.) Nipple shields, which should be banned, are referred to by lactation experts as the kiss of death for breastfeeding.

Creams and Ointments

Since the first edition of this book was published, more information has come to light about sore, dry, or cracked nipples. The cream Lansinoh—an ultra purified, single ingredient, modified lanolin cream endorsed by La Leche League—is now recommended. Lansinoh has no allergenic components and can be applied to the entire nipple area. Since nipples are, afterall, skin, moisturizing them when they are dry helps to speed up healing and prevent scab formation. Other breastfeeding books and the previous edition of this book provided suggestions for combatting this problem by air drying or using your own breastmilk as relief. These methods are now discouraged.

Nursing Pads

You may need nursing pads to absorb milk leakage, but not all nursing pads are created equal. If you buy nursing pads that do *not* have the following features, you're counting on an irritation or a yeast infection.

Look for these features when shopping for nursing pads:

- All-cotton or all-paper pads, which allow maximum air circulation.
- White rather than colored pads (colored pads may contain dyes that will irritate your breasts).
- Pads that are large enough to effectively absorb the milk.

Don't go anywhere near nursing pads that boast:

- A plastic or waterproof lining to trap wetness (these keep the air from getting to your nipples and cause the pad to stick to your skin).
- Synthetic materials (these will prevent air circulation).
- Pretty colors (dyes can irritate the skin around the breast and armpit).

Remember that nursing pads that don't breathe invite yeast infections (or thrush), which live and grow in the milk absorbed in the pads. As an alternative to this messy business, you can learn to shut off your letdown (I'll tell you how in chapter 4); in the meantime, folded tissues, hankies, or cut-up cloth diapers, sheets, and so on work just fine.

Even if you have purchased high-quality nursing pads, it's a good idea to wash your hands after handling the used pads and to change your pads after every feeding.

IF YOU'RE ANTICIPATING PROBLEMS

While it's difficult to predict many breastfeeding problems until feeding actually begins, some women know by now whether they are likely to have a difficult time. For example, it will be obvious to you before you get pregnant if you have inverted or flat nipples. If they don't pop out spontaneously (as most do) during pregnancy, this will be apparent by the third trimester. Or if you've had breast augmentation or reduction surgery, you know that you are at risk for producing a low milk supply.

Hypolactation

It's important to know if you're at risk for poor milk production, known as *hypolactation* (hypo means "too little"). The following are some telltale signs:

- Breasts that don't enlarge during pregnancy and/or don't get sore in the first trimester.
- Unusually shaped breasts, especially those that have very little mammary tissue you can feel.
- History of previous breast surgery, such as breast reduction, reconstruction, or augmentation. (If the milk ducts were cut, hypolactation usually results.)
- History of low milk production with a previous pregnancy. Unless the problem can be identified and fixed (which often happens), odds are that your previous history will repeat itself.
- History of postpartum hemorrhage (this may interfere with your pituitary gland's abililty to produce adequate amounts of prolactin).

What Should You Do?

Prior to delivery, make sure that you see a lactation consultant and voice your concerns. You and your LC can put together some realistic backup plans that range from supplementing your breast milk with a feeder using donated milk or formula, to taking a lactagogue medication, which stimulates breast milk production. Supplementing is discussed in detail in chapter 6.

Preparing Inverted or Flat Nipples

The anatomical realities and challenges of inverted and flat nipples are discussed in chapter 1. Most inverted nipples correct themselves spontaneously as the pregnancy progresses, but flat nipples tend to stay flat. If an inverted nipple does not correct itself, or if you have a flat nipple, a new product called Evert-It™ from Maternal Concepts™ can help draw them out. The product is a soft, plungerlike device available from La Leche League International (see the appendix) or by calling the manufacturer directly at 1-800-310-5817. Breast shells should not be used. The previous edition of this book presented exercises, such as the Hoffman Technique and nipple rolls, but new evidence suggests that these exercises may be harmful.

chapter 4

The First Week of Breastfeeding

Have you ever witnessed the birth of a mammal on one of those nature shows? Has your cat ever had kittens, or dog ever had puppies? Did you grow up on a farm? Inevitably, whether these scenes come to us via television or experience, we marvel at how instinct plays such a huge role in a newborn mammal's survival. Be it kitten or giraffe, the mother immediately begins to lick off the membranes from the newborn, cleaning out its nose and eyes. In some cases, the mother eats her own placenta and then regurgitates it into the newborn's mouth for nourishment. But amazingly, whether the newborn is blind at first (typical for most mammals), forced to recover from a six-foot fall (as the newborn giraffe must), or obligated to deal with an enormous drop in temperature (as an Arctic baby seal must), the newborn immediately begins to search for its mother's nipple and always begins feeding minutes after birth. In some circumstances, if the newborn doesn't find the nipple within a certain time, it will starve or the mother may not allow the nursling to suckle. In other circumstances, the mother mammal positions herself in such a way as to facilitate easy locating of the nipple.

Human babies are no different from their mammal cousins. They, too, must begin feeding immediately in order to survive. Unfortunately, years of humans meddling with the birth process has resulted in us forgetting that we have a breastfeeding instinct, too. So, if we didn't interfere with a newborn human, he would make his way from birth up the mother's stomach to the breast and would start to nurse without any help. But in our current society, breastfeeding for humans isn't automatic, like breathing. It is a skill that both the mother and baby have to acquire.

The first week of breastfeeding is the most difficult week. Too many women give up on breastfeeding at this time because of poor counseling or not enough information. But know this: the longer you breastfeed, the easier it gets. If you have problems getting started, don't panic. Almost all problems can be prevented or fixed—which is why I am devoting an entire chapter to this first, critical week. Everything you need to know about getting started with breastfeeding is here: positioning, latching, milk letdown, pitfalls, common problems, and solutions—plus complete sections on feeding abnormally shaped mouths, more than one baby, and after a cesarean section. (Information on breastfeeding a premature newborn is discussed in chapter 6, and engorgement and painful nursing is discussed in chapter 7.)

It's also worthwhile filling out the questionnaire on page 127. If you're unhappy with your hospital's performance on the baby-friendly scale, do as the questionnaire instructs, and send it to your hospital's administrator.

THE ASAP RULE

As discussed in chapter 3, if you've put breastfeeding on your birth plan, you should be able to begin feeding as soon as the baby's health signs are pronounced strong. Feeding as soon as possible and as often and as long as the baby wants will prevent engorgement, which is when your breasts become swollen and overfilled with milk. Immediate feeding at delivery also speeds up the delivery of the placenta and helps to control blood loss, since the suckling causes the uterus to contract.

Babies also tend to be more alert and interested in feeding in the first hour following birth than even later that day. That's why ASAP is the best rule to follow. If you've had a difficult delivery and need to recover for a few hours, even holding the baby close will help stimulate milk production. If your baby is sick or in intensive care, begin to express your milk immediately to get the process started.

You will not be producing milk until at least two days after delivery. Instead, the baby will be nourished by your colostrum, an incredibly rich source of nutrients replete with anti-infective properties.

Since not all newborns instinctively know how to suckle, you have to *show* them by having what amounts to a "breast rehearsal." Unfortunately, many new mothers aren't aware of this, so when their initial breastfeeding attempts are not successful, they feel as though their breasts just "weren't made for suckling." As a result, many just give up and decide that bottle-feeding is the only route. This is a most unfortunate choice, having more to do with poor lactation *counseling* than poor lactation.

Be patient: Several days of bumbling breastfeeding attempts are the rule, not the exception. Almost every woman *can* breastfeed, but some women face more obstacles than others. With the appropriate instruction, most mothers who want to breastfeed will be able to. Read on to get off to the right start.

Getting into Position

There isn't one set breastfeeding position. Every woman will find different positions comfortable at different stages of breastfeeding. For the very first feeding, it helps to be *shown* a position before you begin to experiment.

Positioning is crucial to getting started. The right position will make it easier for the baby to learn to suckle well, which will ensure a good milk supply and will also help prevent the sore nipples that result from a poor latch. Once you've found a comfortable feeding position, learning the right "latch" technique (discussed shortly) is vital.

Cradle-Hold Position

For this most common daytime position, sit up in bed or in a comfortable chair. As an option, put pillows behind your back to support your muscles, under your elbow on your nursing side, and on your lap (at least until the baby is bigger) to support and raise the baby to your chest level. A stool for your feet will also do the trick. That way you don't need to lean over the baby, which can give you a backache, and even cause shooting pains in the breast itself. Such discomfort interferes with the latch and could lead to sore nipples. Bring the baby's weight onto your chest or onto the pillow(s) in your lap so that the baby-supporting arm doesn't tire.

Hold the baby firmly in your arms, the base of the head in the crook of your arm with baby's back supported by your forearm, and buttocks or thighs cupped by your hand.

Position the baby on her side with her stomach pulled in close to yours. The baby should not have to turn her head to grasp the breast.

If you're in a pinch and don't have any pillows, use a diaper bag, folded coat, and so on.

Lying Down

This is a common position for nighttime feedings. Lie on your side and have your baby facing you on his side, directly at your breast, putting a pillow behind him for support. To change sides, sit the baby up, burp him, then lie flat on your back, holding the baby. This is a particularly good position if you're recovering from a cesarean section or have flat nipples. You can place pillows under your head for support. Your body should be at an angle to the bed as you lean slightly backward into another pillow placed behind your back. An optional third pillow can be placed between your bent knees to elevate your top leg while placing it over and slightly in front of your bottom leg. The baby's head rests in the crook of your arm, as in the cradle hold, or flat on the bed.

Football Hold

Here you're in a sitting position, the baby's legs under your arm and along your sides with her head resting in the hand of that arm. Make sure that the baby's legs aren't pushing up against the back of the chair. If they are, bend the legs so that the baby's rear end is against the chair.

As for pillows, they're placed at your side and even on your lap to raise the baby up to the level of your breast. A pillow behind your shoulders may help you relax (if it doesn't keep falling down!). The baby's bottom rests on the pillow near your elbow.

This position works well if you have large breasts or flat nipples, if you've had a cesarean delivery, or if your baby is sleepy and is experiencing difficulty in learning to breastfeed. (Sleepy babies are discussed toward the end of this chapter, on page 116.)

If your arm gets tired, you can support your forearm with your thigh by bending your knee and placing your foot on a footstool or coffee table. An extra pillow or folded blanket can also help to support your wrist and hand under the baby's head.

If you're feeding multiples, you'll be using the "double football hold" position, discussed on page 114 farther on.

Transitional Hold (aka Modified Cradle Hold)

This is the same as the cradle hold, but the baby's head is in the hand of the opposite arm (rather than in the crook of the same arm you're using to hold the baby). If you're sitting up to feed, this is the position you can use when you switch feeding from one breast to the other. In the transitional hold, unlike the cradle hold, you'll need to put a hand behind the baby's head for support instead of using the crook of your elbow. This gives you better control of the baby's head and is especially important for a premie (who tends to roll up in a ball when the cradle hold is used) or a baby with low muscle tone, a weak rooting reflex, or a weak suck, who will be able to stay on the breast more easily by gently supporting the back of the head.

For a proper transitional hold, the baby and pillows are exactly the same as a cradle hold (see above), but you hold the baby's head with the arm opposite to the offered breast. For example, if you're breastfeeding on your left breast, you'll support the baby's head with your right hand and use your left hand to support your breast. On the right side, you'd use your left hand to support the baby's head and the right hand to support the breast.

If You're Large-Breasted

The football hold is often a good choice here. If you choose to lie down, you can feed from your lower breast first and then bend over the baby to nurse him from the other breast without having to roll over yourself. Or you can try to roll over to the other side with the baby lying on your chest. (This will often help bring up a burp, too.)

Latching On

Even with a good position, a bad latch spells P-A-I-N. Here are step-by-step instructions to a good latch (see figure 4-1):

Step 1: Tummy to tummy. Once you're in a comfortable position (many women prefer to have the head of a bed cranked up, particularly after a

Figure 4-1
GOOD LATCH AND POOR LATCH

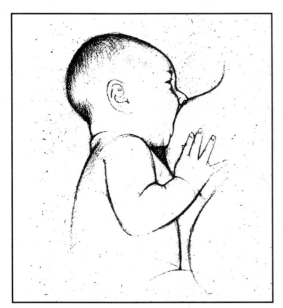

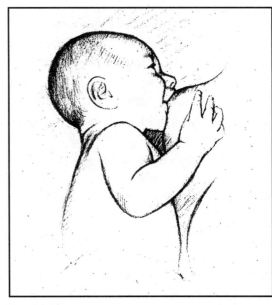

Good latch.   Poor latch.

Illustrations by Karen Visser © 1998.

C-section), position your baby with tummy to yours, her body horizontal. If you like, you can manually pull out your nipple (with your thumb and index finger) so that it is erect.

Step 2: Nose to nipple.   The baby's nose should be level with your nipple. Support your breast by holding four fingers underneath, away from the areola, with your thumb on the nipple (known as the "c-hold"). *Bring your baby to your breast rather than the breast to the baby.*

Step 3: Tickle 'til wide open mouth.   Arouse your baby's sense of taste and smell by expressing a few drops of milk. Now take the nipple and lightly brush it against the baby's lips. This will get the baby interested and may trigger the instinct to suckle. It will also make the nipple erect. Do this until the baby opens his mouth WIDE (as in a yawn). Aim the nipple into the center of the baby's mouth and pop baby onto the breast. *You may need to re-*

peat this step several times before you can move on to step 4. Move onto step 4 only after the baby takes the nipple into its mouth. Do *not* force the nipple in; if you do, the baby will take in only the tip of the nipple, causing a bad latch and pain.

Step 4: Pop baby on!   Very crucial: *Make sure that the baby takes the areola into her mouth along with the nipple.* If just the nipple goes in, you will quickly develop soreness and cracking. Remember, it is the *areola* that contains the milk storage space (sinuses). Unless this is being compressed when the baby suckles, your milk-delivery system won't work effectively. When you see the baby open wide, pop the baby's head toward your breast quickly, which will encourage a better mouthful and help the baby's tongue and lips close in the right position. The nipple should touch the roof of the mouth toward the back of the baby's throat. This stimulates effective suckling and enables the baby's gums to compress the milk sinuses on the areola. When the breast is far enough back in the baby's mouth, the nipple is also protected from being gummed or chewed. If the nipple is *not* touching the roof of the mouth, the baby may turn her head back and forth in confusion. If this happens, put your finger in the corner of the baby's mouth, break the suction, take the baby off the breast, and repeat this step.

Step 5: Check the latch.   Your baby is latched on properly if the mouth is widely open around the breast; the tip of the tongue is above the lower lip and is cradled around your nipple; and the nose is just touching the breast. In addition, the jaw should move up and down, the ears should wiggle, and the nipple should feel *comfortable.* Cheeks should *not* be sucking in and out as they do with bottle-feeding.

Step 6: Ignore all feeding schedules.   Nurse the baby as long as possible, as often as possible. In other words, *no schedules.* Feed the baby from both sides as much as he wants, for as long as he wants. This means at least eight to ten times per twenty-four hours for the first week of life.

Step 7: Help baby off.   When your baby's "full" and has clearly stopped feeding, don't pull out the nipple yet. Break the suction by inserting a finger into the corner of the baby's mouth. This will let in some air and help the baby let go. It will also be a lot easier on your nipple. (There are other techniques to break the suction too, but this is the best way.)

Women who learn to position their babies close enough to the breast to ensure a good latch early on should experience only minimal nipple soreness or tenderness as nursing progresses. A poor latch is the most common reason for sore nipples and pain during nursing. See chapter 7 for all the details.

If You Need to Stop Feeding Mid-Nursing

If you have to take the baby off your breast before he is finished, just break the suction as discussed above.

My Baby Won't "Open Wide"

To get the baby to open her mouth wide like a yawn, try saying "open" as you tickle the baby's lips with your nipple. Some babies respond better if you lightly tickle the bottom lip only. Eventually, the baby will learn to associate the word *open* with opening her mouth wide and being rewarded with the breast.

If the baby's mouth remains closed or doesn't open wide enough, be patient and keep repeating "open" while tickling the baby's lips with your nipple. Most babies will learn to open wide. If necessary, you can open the baby's mouth wider by gently but firmly pushing down on the lower lip with the index finger of the hand supporting the breast.

As a last resort, you can stimulate the baby's gag reflex in order to get her to open wide, but this will not work if the baby becomes frustrated. In fact, she might begin to associate gagging with nursing—the last thing you want. So if it seems to bother your baby, this is probably not a good method.

My Baby Isn't "Popping On"

If you're having trouble bringing the baby to your breast, you may not be moving fast enough. You have to move really quickly once you see that wide-open mouth. In one rapid motion, bring your baby onto your breast using the same arm that's actually holding the baby. This is often easier with the transitional hold than the regular cradle hold. Bring the weight of your baby's body onto your chest rather than leaning over the baby.

Great—But Can My Baby Breathe?

If you're worried, make sure that the baby is tucked around your middle horizontally so he can breathe out the sides of his nose no matter how close he is to the breast. To create more of an airway, try pulling your baby's bottom in closer, and drop your shoulder down on the side that's being nursed. This will lower the baby's head in relation to the rest of his body.

Or lift up your breast from underneath. This will also give the baby more of an airway. As the baby matures and the suck becomes stronger, you may not need to do this if you're small- to medium-breasted, but large-breasted women avoid buckling, which can trigger conditions such as mastitis or plugged ducts (see chapter 7).

Finally, if the baby's nose seems to be blocked by the breast, lift up your breast and either drop your shoulder or pull the baby's legs and body in closer to you. This is better than pressing down on the top of the breast. (Your positioning may also need some adjusting once you do this.)

My Baby Can't Seem to Grasp My Nipples

If the baby has difficulty grasping the breast, you may be slightly engorged. In this case, express a little milk prior to feeding to soften the breast. Even if you have a flat nipple, a baby can pull it up without a problem so long as you're not engorged.

How Do I Get My Nipples to Protrude?

It's helpful to use an erect nipple to tickle the baby's lips and get her mouth to open. If caressing the nipple isn't enough, do a few nipple pulls (discussed in chapter 3) prior to feeding. If that doesn't work, place your fingers on your breast about an inch behind the edge of the areola. With your thumb above and your index finger below, push the skin of the breast back toward the chest wall as the baby latches on.

If they still don't protrude, try pressing a moist cold cloth over the nipple *only,* and then blow on it or use the syringe trick discussed in chapter 3.

I Can't Seem to Maintain My Position!

Here's a huge hint: If you're not in a comfortable position from the moment that mouth hits your nipple, it's not as easy to keep the breast properly positioned in your baby's mouth. Without support, your arm muscles can get really tired, and the baby then drops down below the breast. This pulls the breast forward in the baby's mouth, and his jaws start chewing the nipple, causing soreness. That's why all those pillows, towels, and footstools can be so helpful.

To determine whether you're in the right position (for cradle hold or lying down), here's what should be happening:

1. You're comfortable with your arms and back supported.

2. You are not leaning over the baby.

3. In the cradle hold, the baby is "chest to chest," knees to your other breast.

4. Your baby's stomach is pulled in close to yours.

5. Your baby's ear, shoulder, and hip are in a straight line.

6. You hold your breast with your thumb on top and fingers underneath.

When the baby begins nursing, here's what you should see:

1. The chin and the tip of the baby's nose touch (or almost touch) your breast during the entire nursing.

2. The baby's lips are flanged out and relaxed.

3. The baby's tongue is cupped below the breast. (You can gently pull down on the baby's lower lip to check.)

4. You notice a "wiggle" at the baby's temple and ear while she nurses.

5. Once your milk has let down, you hear swallowing after every one or two suckles for five to ten minutes on each side at each feeding. By the end of the feeding, swallows may follow every four or five sucks.

I Think My Breasts Are Too Big for My Baby!

Just because your breasts are large doesn't mean that your nipples are. I promise: Your baby will *not* suffocate when you pull him close to nurse. In fact, your baby's pug nose is designed to allow for breathing from the sides.

If you're large-breasted, support your breast from underneath and put only as much areola and breast as your hand can hold toward the baby's mouth. Then support your breast with your hand, a tiny pillow, or rolled-up towels during the entire feeding to keep the weight of your breast from pulling the nipple out of the baby's mouth.

Some women find the football hold to be easiest while the baby learns to breastfeed during the first weeks.

If you're nursing lying down, you don't need to support your breasts at all. Just place the baby at a slight angle to your body, get her latched on, and then pull her legs in close to you. You can roll toward the baby to nurse from the top breast.

In public, good positions are the cradle hold, the transitional hold, the football hold, and sitting cross-legged on the floor with the baby's head on a pillow in your lap rather than in the crook of your arm.

What If I Have a Really Big Areola?

The average areola has a radius of about one to one and a half inches from the nipple to the edge. If your areola's circumference is larger than this, just offer as much as the baby's mouth can accommodate. Nursing will go just fine. Most newborns can't take *any* complete areola into their mouths, no matter what size it is.

Do I Still Need to Support My Breast If I'm Small-Breasted?

No. If your breast isn't sagging, there's no need to support it. But if your breasts begin to feel tender once you begin nursing, it might help. The more your baby suckles, the more milk your breasts will make, which may increase their size slightly. In general, though, it is fat, not glandular, tissue that causes women's breasts to differ in size.

ALL ABOUT LETDOWN

After the first two to three days of good breastfeeding positioning and latch, your milk will begin to "come in" and will replace the colostrum that your newborn has been feeding on thus far. (If your latch and positioning have been unsuccessful or you haven't been nursing often enough or long enough, when your milk comes in you will experience engorgement, discussed on page 175 in chapter 7.) Your milk "coming in" is *not* to be confused with milk "letdown," which occurs when your myoepithelial cells actively squeeze the milk out of the breast into the milk sinuses. Milk letdown is also called the "letdown reflex" or the "milk-ejection reflex."

What happens during letdown is that while some milk accumulates in the milk reservoirs behind the nipple and in the ducts, most of the milk is made and stored in other parts of the breast. The letdown reflex releases this milk into the milk ducts, making it available to the baby.

The baby's suckling stimulates the letdown. The rhythmic motion of jaws, lips, and tongue send nerve impulses to your pituitary gland, which releases oxytocin.

Some women first experience milk letdown when they're not even feeding, and may notice milk dripping from their breasts after a shower, for example. The milk literally flows out of the nipple and may even spray outward. A baby who is at the breast when this happens will happily gulp down the milk (unless you have an overactive letdown, discussed presently). If this happens when you're not feeding, you can shut off the letdown.

Learning to Let Down

One of the reasons it takes a couple of days for your letdown reflex to get going is because the reflex has to be developed. As your baby suckles, the milk flows from the milk glands, where it is produced, to beneath the nipple, where it sprays right down the baby's throat. If the baby has not latched on properly, letdown may not occur. As discussed in chapter 1, once the suckling begins, it sets off an entire hormonal symphony that triggers milk production.

So because letdown is a reflex that must be acquired, the more you nurse, the more efficient your body becomes at letting down your milk when your baby nurses. If you stop nursing before letdown occurs, only a third of the milk in the breast is available to your baby. This means that the baby will not only receive less milk but will be denied any of the higher-calorie hind-milk, which clings to the ducts and is available to the baby only with letdown.

In the first few weeks of breastfeeding, assuming your latch and positioning are good, it takes anywhere from five to fifteen minutes of nursing for letdown to occur. Once you've hung in there and become a real pro, letdown will occur within a minute or two of nursing. There are usually a number of letdowns with each nursing, but the first is always the strongest.

When Your Letdown Is Slowed Down

Breast hormones are no different from other female hormones; they slow down when you're under stress. Just as you might miss your period when you're under tension or stress, your breast hormones may also slow down milk production if you're stressed. This slowing down is what some refer to as a "prehistoric" instinct that kicks in when reproduction of the species seems "threatened." When your Neanderthal predecessors were, say, running from an attacking tribe or man-eating beast, their breasts would *not* be dripping with milk!

Outside factors that contribute to a delayed letdown are tension, stress, fatigue, anxiety, physical pain (often caused by a bad latch or poor position), smoking, excessive alcohol, and some drugs. If you suspect stress and tension are to blame, you might want to discuss with your doctor or LC the possibility of seeking counseling.

If you smoke or take in too much alcohol, try cutting out these vices and see if your letdown improves. If you're on certain medications that are affecting your letdown, discuss finding a substitute medication that will not interfere. (See chapter 3 for more details.)

If the letdown is delayed or inhibited, the baby may nurse well for a few minutes and then pull away in frustration. You may also notice that your baby is sucking rapidly but not *swallowing* as much as he should be. In this case, the baby will get only the milk that has accumulated in the milk reservoirs near the nipple; without the letdown reflex, most of your milk will remain inside the breast despite the baby's efforts. A poor letdown is another common cause of soreness during nursing, further discussed in the Common Problems section at the end of this chapter.

What Does Letdown Feel Like?

Here are some common signs that indicate your letdown reflex is working just fine. Most women will experience at least some of the following:

- Tingling sensations or a feeling of fullness, particularly at the beginning of each feeding. At the beginning, some women may find this uncomfortable and, if they are engorged, quite painful. But the feeding will empty the breast, and the discomfort associated with this sensation will fade as the baby gets older. Some women describe this as a "pins-and-needles" or achy feeling.

- Leaking from the other breast while nursing.

- Leaking when thinking about your baby or hearing the baby cry.

- Uterine cramping ("afterpains") while you're nursing. That's your oxytocin going to work. The cramping is a sign that your uterus is shrinking down to its normal size. Afterpains will stop after the first two weeks of feeding. They tend to become more pronounced with each subsequent baby.

- Feeling of relaxation or well-being. That's your prolactin going to work, which actually helps to relax you and improves your mood, even causing a sense of euphoria.

- Changes in baby's suckling pattern during feeding. Once the milk comes in, the baby's suckling slows because she has to swallow. With just colostrum, the pattern will go something like: suck suck suck... swallow. (It's a single beat for each suck). After the milk letdown reflex kicks in, you'll hear something like: suck swallow suck swallow. If you listen carefully, you'll notice that there are several letdowns per feed, and the first one will be more like a suckle GULP suckle GULP.

- Milk appearing in the corner of the baby's mouth.

The breast will become soft when it has been well emptied. You can tell when a baby has finished a breast by one or more of the following signs:

- The baby becomes totally relaxed, opens his mouth slightly, and slides off the breast in a state of bliss. If you still need to empty side two, this is the time to switch.

- After a period of lots of sucking and not much swallowing, the baby comes off the breast and fusses, or comes off the breast and yells for more (and the breast is soft).

- The baby is sucking strongly, swallowing very infrequently, and letdown has already occurred several times. In addition, the breast is soft, and the last letdown was some time ago.

How Do You Shut It Off?

Have you ever seen a woman suddenly cross her arms across her chest? Chance are, she's shutting off her milk letdown, which may have been triggered from the cry of a baby or even thoughts about her own child. This letdown reflex may persist for years after her last child has been weaned, until it eventually fades away.

Letdown can be shut off on one or both breasts by pressing firmly with the heel of the hands or the forearms directly over the nipple(s) you want to "turn off." This can be used to stop one side from leaking when nursing on the side.

Letdown Foreplay

In the same way that sexual foreplay, in the form of fantasies, visual images, and touching of certain erogenous zones will trigger "vaginal letdown" (sexual secretions for intercourse), a "foreplay" routine can be practiced that will help to trigger *milk* letdown. (Once the reflex is well established, it will work anywhere, anytime!) Assuming your position is comfortable and your latch technique is correct, try some of the following to help train your reflex:

1. Nurse in a quiet spot away from distractions.

2. Prolong that "tummy to tummy" time. Cuddle and nuzzle with the baby, and smell that wonderful newborn scent.

3. Prior to nursing, relax as much as you can, using whatever works. Whether it's watching old Mary Tyler Moore reruns or practicing yogic breathing techniques, do it!

4. Apply warm compresses to a part of your body before feedings.

5. Massage your breasts and manually stimulate your nipples before feedings (your partner can do this for you too).

6. Think good "baby" thoughts.

7. Turn on the faucet to help trigger thoughts of running water and milk flowing.

8. If you've been pumping to keep up your milk supply, sometimes just turning on the pump prior to feeding will get your milk flowing.

BREASTFEEDING AFTER A C-SECTION

A cesarean section may limit your comfort in terms of positioning, but the baby's sucking will stimulate your uterus to contract more quickly, speeding up your healing.

Not all cesarean mothers will experience the same breastfeeding challenges. Women who have had an epidural or spinal anesthetic will be able to begin nursing shortly after delivery. Those who've had a general anesthetic, however, might experience a bit more of a delay, since they'll need some time to come out of the anesthetic. In this case, holding the baby close and cuddling can begin right after coming to, and breastfeeding can begin shortly thereafter.

If any supplementing is medically necessary while you're still unconscious, it should be in the form of banked breast milk or formula (not water or sugar water) from a cup or feeding tube—not a bottle. (See chapter 6.) Your partner or support person should make this clear to the hospital staff on your behalf.

The Emotional "Letdown"

Because you've had major abdominal surgery, your hospital and postpartum experience will differ from that of your vaginal-birth peers. Your hospital stay is usually longer, you're in more discomfort, you may not be able to have rooming-in privileges (depending on hospital policies), and you may be more dependent on hospital staff. In fact, before you experience milk letdown, you'll most likely be dealing with some emotional letdown first.

The usual hospital stay after a cesarean section is about four days if both you and the baby are doing well. But whatever the length of stay, try to arrange for some help around the house via your partner, mother, or friends to help you get your energy back faster and to enable you to concentrate on getting a good start with breastfeeding.

If you've had an unexpected cesarean, you may be feeling "robbed" of that childbirth experience you were so looking forward to. This can affect your ability to breastfeed, since you may feel detached from your baby. You may resent the baby on some level for being "too big" or turned the wrong way. You may also be just plain p.o.'d at your doctor for choosing to do a cesarean (even if it was indicated). All these feelings can easily get mixed in with general maternal blues.

What Should You Do?

Let people know how you feel; holding in your feelings will only exacerbate the problem. Ask to spend some time with an LC or hospital social worker or counselor. Also begin to hold your baby close ASAP. Touching and holding your baby will help to comfort you, because the smell of the baby and feel of her will help to physically trigger your milk hormones.

If the cesarean was planned, you probably won't experience this kind of emotional upheaval, because you will have had some time to adjust to the idea, and to make certain provisions on your birth plan to facilitate ASAP breastfeeding.

Is Your Hospital Baby-Friendly?

As discussed in chapter 3, there is currently a global effort to initiate the ten steps to baby-friendly hospitals, but many hospitals are not there yet, and their policies can sometime interfere with breastfeeding. To combat some of these rules, request the following from hospital staff:

1. No artificial nipples. (See Confused about "Nipple Confusion" farther on.)

2. For a planned cesarean, request to be kept with the baby after birth if you're both healthy (some hospitals and doctors require a mandatory observation period in the nursery for all babies born by cesarean).

3. Twenty-four-hour rooming-in privileges. Keep in mind that rooming-in hours vary widely from hospital to hospital.

4. Dad rooming in to help you, if baby is rooming in. (This may not be possible, but it doesn't hurt to ask.)

If your hospital or birthing facility requires that the baby be observed for twenty-four hours, and if you can't get the baby to room in with you, INSIST, unless he's ill, that the baby be brought to you for all feedings. If you're separated from the baby due to health problems, begin to express your colostrum as soon as possible and have it fed to the baby with one of the techniques discussed in chapter 6. Then, at all possible junctures, try to breastfeed when you and the baby are together.

If you need to be on medication, make sure it's compatible with breastfeeding. As discussed in chapter 3, substitute medications can usually be used in the event of a conflict.

Finding a Position

Finding a comfortable position after a cesarean section can be a challenge. Your best bet is the lying-down position, discussed on page 90. In this case, however, you should place a pillow between the baby's feet and your incision. This pillow can also be tucked under your abdomen to support the sagging muscles, whose ligaments, supporting your uterus, could get stretched, thereby causing further discomfort. To roll over and minimize pulling your stitches, use your leg muscles to scoot your hips over to the other side.

Feeding on the Delivery Table

If you begin to breastfeed on the delivery table, you may need to nurse while lying on your back. If you've had a spinal anesthetic, you'll need to lie flat to prevent a spinal headache. Some other challenges may arise if one or both arms are restrained or if an intravenous tube is still in place.

In this case, you may be able to turn to one side and breastfeed in a side-lying position (lying-down position) once your incision is closed. Your partner or nurse can help you get the baby into position and arrange pillows for your comfort. (If pillows are not available, your partner can physically support you while you nurse.)

Feeding with an IV

If your IV is inserted into the back of your hand, it may restrict your movements and make it more difficult to find a comfortable nursing position. A supporting piece of cardboard attached to your hand can help keep your IV in place without interfering with breastfeeding.

You can also ask for your IV drip to be transferred to your forearm with extra tape to secure the IV tubing.

If You're Not Feeling Well

Because you've had pelvic surgery, it's possible to develop an infection at the incision site (bacteria got into the incision), a pelvic infection (bacteria can enter your open pelvis), or even a urinary tract infection (from the catheter following surgery). Any of these infections can be accompanied by fever, pain, or discomfort.

If you have an infection, as long as your hands are clean before you touch the baby, there's no reason to be separated.

If you're on pain medication or antibiotics, make sure the drugs are compatible with breastfeeding. (See chapter 3.)

CONFUSED ABOUT "NIPPLE CONFUSION"?

Nipple confusion is a poorly worded, overtechnical term that winds up confusing women and newborns even *more*. In other words, most of the material available on the subject is simply too confusing for the average person to comprehend!

In order to understand exactly what nipple confusion really is, please erase this awful phrase and replace it with "real nipples versus fake nipples." Simpler, isn't it? To a newborn, there is a world of difference between real nipples and rubber nipples. With real nipples the baby suckles; with rubber nipples, the baby *sucks*. So when you're first teaching the baby how to breast-feed, and you're working hard to get all that positioning and latching correct, it doesn't make a lot of sense to introduce a new and different nipple, does it? That's basically all there is to "nipple confusion."

To find out what it is about fake nipples that confuse a breastfeeding baby so much, read on.

Sucking vs. Suckling

For every action required by the mouth and tongue in suckling, there is an equal, opposite reaction required by the mouth when sucking. Hence, sucking is an entirely different technique from suckling. If you teach the suckling baby to *suck* too early on, she may never go back to suckling again.

Since it's probably been a while since you had your last bottle, here's what your mouth does when it sucks from a rubber nipple, be it bottle or pacifier:

1. To grasp the rubber nipple, the mouth does not need to open wide. The lips close around the small rubber nipple. Get a baby used to this, and you can kiss breastfeeding good-bye, because the baby will grasp less of the breast and chomp down on the nipple, thereby causing sore nipples and missing the areola altogether, which means not emptying the breast properly.

2. The mouth engages far less jaw action with rubber nipples than real ones. (In breastfeeding, the jaw action is what draws out the milk!)

3. The tongue presses hard up against the inflexible rubber nipple. In breastfeeding, the tongue only cradles the nipple. A rubber-nipple tongue-thrust habit will rub a real nipple raw.

4. With rubber nipples, milk drips into the mouth as the bottle is held higher. So a baby returning to the breast will not understand why the milk doesn't flow immediately.

Few babies are able to master the technique of sucking *and* suckling until they are at least two or three months old and breastfeeding well. It's akin to learning bicycling and skateboarding simultaneously.

Questions?

Q. How many rubber nipples does it take to confuse a baby?
A. One. Especially in the early weeks.

Q. Are some babies more "confusable" than others?
A. Sleepy babies and babies with a weak suck are more susceptible to becoming confused than babies who take the breast without any difficulty.

Q. When can I give my baby a bottle or pacifier?
A. Lactation experts recommend waiting anywhere from four to six weeks before introducing rubber nipples. This will give the baby time to learn how to breastfeed properly.

Q. What if I need to supplement my breast milk?
A. If this is necessary in the first four to six weeks, review chapter 6 for more details.

Q. What products are considered rubber nipples?
A. Bottles, pacifiers, and nipple shields (which should be banned).

Q. Is there any hope of breastfeeding if you have already introduced rubber nipples to your baby?
A. Don't worry; you're not doomed, but you will need to spend some time retraining your baby to accept your breast. If this is the case, discuss your situation with a lactation consultant, and work out a *realistic* retraining plan with her. This will include pumping your breasts to keep up your breast-milk supply so the baby can actually get milk on beginning breastfeeding again.

THE MOUTHS OF BABES

Not all babies have the same kind of mouth. For example, some babies have a weaker suck, while others can have low muscle tone or even a short tongue. Still others are tongue-tied or have a cleft lip or palate. As a result, some babies have more difficulty latching on and staying on the breast.

If your baby has one of these anatomical variations, you may not be able to nurse effectively using the common nursing positions discussed earlier in the chapter. Instead, you'll need to consult your baby's doctor or pediatrician or an LC and adjust your position to accommodate the baby's facial structure. Often, the right positioning can make it possible to nurse a baby with a receding chin, high and/or narrow arch in the palate, cleft lip, cleft palate, short tongue, and so on.

Nursing a Cleft-Palate Baby

Babies with a cleft palate can't suckle very effectively on their own because they can't hold the nipple at the back of the mouth the way other babies can. They can, however, "milk" the breast with their gums and tongue when the breast is very full, which enables them to hold onto the breast better.

Your best bet is to place your index finger on the top edge of your areola, keeping your middle finger on the bottom. Then press your nipple out between your two fingers so that it protrudes the way it would if it were full of milk. Use your other fingers to lift the breast into the baby's mouth. This way, your baby will get the letdown milk. You'll then need to hold your nipple in during the entire feeding, pressing the baby to the breast throughout.

Surgery to repair the palate is available but isn't usually recommended until the baby is two years of age. In the meantime, your baby can be fitted with an appliance that looks like a top denture without teeth, which will seal the hole in the palate and make nursing easier.

If you're having difficulty with your positioning and latching and find you need to supplement, feed the baby when your breasts are full, pump the excess milk to empty the breast, and feed the baby your expressed milk with a feeding tube. See chapter 6 for more details on supplementing.

Nursing a Baby with a Cleft Lip

This is different from a cleft palate. Cleft-lip babies can breastfeed beautifully, except that you'll probably notice milk leaking out around the cleft lip. Don't worry about this; it won't bother the baby. Make sure that you see an LC or doctor to make sure your position is the best it can be. Then just carry on. Lip surgery is available to fix the cleft anywhere between two weeks and four months of age.

When that happens, what most mothers do is breastfeed their babies normally until two hours prior to surgery. As soon as the baby comes out of the anesthetic, breastfeeding can begin again. This does not interfere with healing, since the suckling stimulates a good blood supply and faster healing for the baby.

If Your Baby Is Tongue-Tied

You can tell if your baby is tongue-tied (or has a short frenulum) when he cries. You'll see that the tongue rises up in a heart shape instead of a smooth curve. This is very easy to fix by having your baby's doctor or pediatrician clip the fold of tissue under the baby's tongue. Until the tissue is clipped, breastfeeding may be more difficult. What you can do is express your milk by pumping until the procedure is done. You can also try to feed your colostrum or milk via feeding tube at the breast (see chapter 6) until the procedure.

A baby who is tongue-tied would be able to suck on a finger or a rubber nipple, but would not be able to cup the breast with his tongue. Curiously, some tongue-tied babies can breastfeed on one breast but not the other.

The Clipping Procedure

Clipping a short frenulum is a simple, in-office procedure. In the past, babies who were not truly tongue-tied had this procedure performed unnecessarily, which gave it a bad name. Fortunately, today only those babies with short frenulums are diagnosed as tongue-tied, and the clipping truly solves their breastfeeding problems.

If you're having trouble finding a doctor willing to clip the baby's frenulum, check with oral surgeons, dentists, ear-nose-throat specialists, and general surgeons, too. A variety of specialists are qualified to do this.

Feeding with a Short Tongue

Sometimes, a baby is born with a short tongue that prevents her from latching on well or causes her to repeatedly lose hold of the breast while nursing. This baby usually continues to lose weight after your milk comes in.

If the baby isn't getting enough milk, you'll need to express your milk as often as your baby would be feeding and supplement with one of the techniques discussed in chapter 6. Usually, the baby outgrows this condition within four to six weeks, at which time you can begin breastfeeding normally.

Feeding the Baby with a Weak Suck

A baby with a weak suck doesn't have a structural problem at work but is having difficulty developing his suckling *skill.* Babies with weak sucks may frequently fall off the breast. You may also notice that milk is leaking out of the baby's mouth, and in extreme cases the baby may even choke on the milk while nursing.

This can be a serious problem for the baby. Here are the steps to follow if you suspect a weak suck:

1. Have your baby's health evaluated to rule out an illness or infection. (See chapter 8 for information on a variety of infant ailments.)

2. See an LC or your baby's doctor to review your positioning and latch-on technique. Experiment with other positions.

3. If, despite a perfect position and latch-on, your baby still cannot stay on the breast, you'll need to review the following:

    - What drugs (if any) you were given during labor and delivery. Your baby may be affected by them.

    - Your baby's "rooting reflex." This suckling reflex should be kicking in naturally. If when you touch one cheek your baby is not moving her head toward the touch, this is a bad sign. Ask your baby's pediatrician or doctor to step in and advise you.

    - Your baby's muscle tone. If your baby is always lying like a rag doll this is a sign of poor muscle tone. In this case, consult a doctor ASAP to rule out a serious illness or neurological impairment. Depending on the cause, it may improve in a few weeks after some decent breastfeeding time. If weak muscle tone is just the way your baby is, consult an LC or your baby's doctor about the best position in this case.

A Catch-22

Unless the suck is improved, the lack of breast stimulation can cause engorgement (see chapter 7), which can affect your milk supply. Then the baby's suck can become even weaker, causing poor weight gain. This causes further deterioration of your milk supply unless you're expressing/pumping your own milk. The problem needs to be corrected fairly soon after birth or your baby may need supplements.

Signs of a Weak Suck

Since it's important to correct this early, here's what to look for if you suspect this problem:

- Nursing for less than five minutes per breast, fewer than eight times in twenty-four hours. Short feedings will occur if the baby tires easily (seen in cardiac or respiratory disease in a baby). One or two shorter feeds are fine, but if this is a continuous pattern in the early days, this won't allow enough time for letdown to occur (you need about fifteen minutes per side at first).

- Fewer than six wet diapers and fewer than two to five stools in twenty-four hours, beginning the day after the milk comes in. (See Is the Customer Satisfied? in chapter 6, page 149.)

What Should You Do?

See your baby's doctor as soon as you recognize the problem. The baby's health should be evaluated to rule out an underlying health problem. In the meantime, expressing/pumping your milk will keep up your milk supply. Then, feed your expressed milk to your baby with a feeding tube or supplement aid until the baby can nurse effectively. If the problem cannot be fixed, this will have to become the norm until you're ready to wean.

To try to get the baby to nurse effectively at the breast, here are some exercises lactation experts recommend:

- Just before feeding, try to gently circle around inside the baby's lips with your index finger three times clockwise, then three times counterclockwise. This may help the baby to get a better seal on the breast.

‽ Just before putting the baby on the breast, touch a clean finger to the tongue for just a moment. This may stimulate the mouth to suckle.

‽ Try the "dancer hand position" to support the baby's chin and hold the jaw steady. This allows the baby to concentrate on nursing. Start by positioning the baby for breastfeeding. Next, rotate the hand you use to support your breast so that your breast rests in the bottom of the "U" formed by your thumb and index finger. Then slide your thumb and index finger forward and in front of your breast, leaving three fingers to support the breast and keep its weight off the baby's chin. Bring the baby close to your breast and support the chin by resting it in the bottom of the U. To steady the baby's jaw, bend your thumb and index finger and gently hold the baby's cheeks while he nurses.

‽ If you haven't already, try the football hold. It works well for babies with a weak suck because it gives you a good view of the baby's face, allowing you to apply gentle pressure to the back of the baby's head, if needed.

MORE THAN A MOUTHFUL

In the past, many doctors discouraged women from breastfeeding more than one baby, fearing poor weight gain and an insufficient milk supply. We now know that this is completely false. The more suckling your breasts receive, *the more milk they'll make.* The rules of latch-on and letdown are exactly the same. In fact, the more the merrier. Breastfeeding your multiples will help get your babies' weights and energies up faster than formula, offering them all the benefits that single babies get from breastfeeding. For very tiny premies, a fortifier may be indicated. While premature breast milk is richer with more calories than term milk, it may not compensate completely for the needs of the very low-birthweight baby.

Just like any new mother who breastfeeds, follow the ASAP rule. If your babies are staying in a neonatal care unit, express your breasts with a pump and have your newborns fed with your colostrum via a feeding tube (discussed more in chapter 6).

The problem with feeding two or more mouths is that you may never get relief from feeding unless you design a feeding/pumping schedule that can provide for some time off. In addition, because your positioning is trickier to coordinate (see below), you of all mothers should *arrange to see a lactation consultant* in your third trimester, or within the first two days of delivery (before engorgement). Also look into joining a breastfeeding peer-support group where you can meet other mothers in your situation. Swapping advice and techniques with other mothers of multiples will go a long way when you're breastfeeding more than one newborn.

One or Two at a Time?

There are advantages to both. Many women find it easier to nurse two babies simultaneously than just one at a time. This rule is fine if both babies take to the breast without difficulty, but if one baby is having difficulty latching on, it's better to give some special attention to training that baby to breastfeed. In this case, one at a time is best. Once the baby catches on, you can feed both babies together again.

Simultaneous nursing triggers a faster, more enhanced letdown, because the suckling from both babies releases higher levels of oxytocin. Nursing two at once won't, of course, necessarily be an option when both babies have different nursing needs and aren't interested in feeding at the same time.

Breastfeeding each baby separately has the advantage of allowing for undivided attention to the nursing baby (although the nursing baby often likes a sibling nearby).

Should I Switch Breasts?

This is an excellent question, and one to which many single-birth mothers can't relate. If you're feeding two babies at a time, and emptying both breasts at the same time, you wouldn't need to switch sides during feeding. So which baby gets which breast . . . and for how long?

Some women simply use the first come, first served approach and offer whichever breast feels most full to whichever baby seems hungriest at the moment. But other mothers actually "reserve" a breast for a particular baby, and keep feeding that baby from that particular breast for the entire day. If this sounds like you, just make sure you give each baby equal time on the left and right breast, alternating breasts, say, each day. Switching breasts will give the babies, quite literally, a different perspective, allowing them to get varied visual stimulation, which they need for their motor development. It is particularly important to switch breasts often for a baby with a weaker suck, for reasons discussed on page 110.

Positioning

First, invest in a large foam nursing pillow, which provides an all-in-one nursing surface for two babies at once. If you'd like to breastfeed two babies at once but are stymied by technical difficulties such as positioning, you'll need to experiment to get it right. That's where an LC or another multiple comrade comes in. Whether you experiment with a variety of pillows or nurse in a bed or a chair, or on a couch or floor, consider these two-at-a-time positions (see also figure 4-2):

- ❧ *Combination cradle and football hold.* You sit upright. One baby is in the cradle hold, while the other is in the football hold with her head on her sibling's abdomen. Pillows under your elbows and the babies make this easier. This is a favored position when you need to nurse away from home, and the easiest one to master if one or both babies have difficulty latching on to the breast.

- ❧ *Criss-cross.* Here you're sitting upright while both babies are in the cradle hold, criss-crossed in your lap. One baby's body is pressed against you, while the other baby's body is pressed against his sibling's. Their heads are in the crooks of your arms. A pillow under your elbow can help support the lower baby.

- ❧ *Parallel.* Sitting upright, your babies' bodies extend in the same direction. One baby is in the cradle hold, with her head in the crook of your arm and her body across your lap. The other baby's body extends in the same direction as his sibling's, off your lap, with his head supported by your hand and arm. Again, this is easier if you use pillows to support your elbows.

- ❧ *Double football hold.* That nursing pillow really comes in handy for this one, which is a variation of the single football hold position, dis-

Figure 4-2
POSITIONING

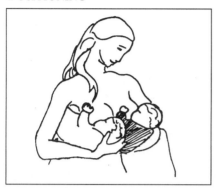

Combination cradle and football hold

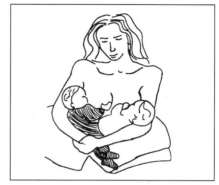

Double cradle hold (criss-cross)

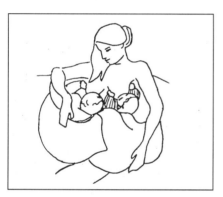

Double football or clutch hold

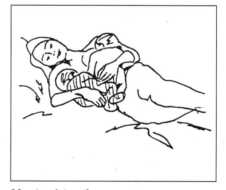

Nursing lying down

Illustrations by Paul Torgus. Reprinted with permission of La Leche League International, 1995.

cussed at the beginning of this chapter. Again, sitting upright, both babies are in the football hold, lying on firm pillows at your sides. The higher the pillows, the kinder this position is to your back. You may also want to prop up your feet on a footstool, chair, or coffee table. If you had your babies by a cesarean section, this position is particularly convenient.

❧ *Stomach.* This is not a very common position because it requires a lot of dexterity on your part. Lie on your stomach and prop yourself up on your elbows. Have the babies lie on their backs underneath you. For the babies, it's a bit like being fed grapes from a doting slave.

Nighttime Nursing

When you have more than one baby on more than one feeding schedule, nighttime nursing can be a nightmare, resulting in virtually no sleep. Fortunately, there are some suggestions for multiple sleeping arrangements that can help you get some sleep.

Many parents of multiples prefer to put two babies in one crib; they find the babies sleep better when they're physically touching one another. Sleeping together also helps synchronize their sleep schedules so *you* get more sleep! This simulates their womb environment. Most women prefer to have the crib in their room so that nighttime nursing involves less motion for you and the babies (they don't rouse as much) and also synchronizes your schedule to theirs.

Some women even fasten the crib to the side of their bed, adjusting the mattress level to theirs and removing the side rail closest to their bed. This provides instant access at night, to facilitate nursing in the side-lying/lying-down position (which doesn't work for simultaneous nursing).

An alternative is for you to sleep on a mattress on the floor (in your room or the babies'), and just sleep with the babies on the floor mattress (so they can't fall off).

Finally, as long as you're careful to build a guard or wall on your own bed, you can just take the babies to bed with you and nurse them on demand. (Do NOT do this if you have a waterbed, or if anyone in your bed is drunk, stoned, or weighs over 300 pounds!)

Don't Play Superwoman

Since you'll be nursing between eight and twelve times every twenty-four hours, you may consider investing in a breast pump (which won't save time until your milk comes in and the extra pumping yields *extra* milk). But when you *can* express/pump extra milk, other family members and friends can then help to feed your babies with that breast milk. You and a lactation consultant can coordinate an agreeable feeding schedule that combines breast feeding and an alternate feeding method that suits you and your babies. (See chapter 5 for more information on expressing/pumping milk and preventing engorgement.) Expressing/pumping will help get your milk supply up faster to feed your babies.

Invest, if at all possible, in a housekeeper, and *accept help* from your partner. Accepting help also means not attempting to be Superwoman and worrying about a messy kitchen or bathroom. If your partner can clean up and share more in the usual household chores, so much the better. But if it becomes a problem, consider lowering your standards for a few months while you and your babies take care of business.

Breastfeeding Triplets or More

Again, since breastfeeding works on supply and demand, the more the merrier. Many women have exclusively breastfed triplets and more until their babies were ready for solids.

Most women will need to express/pump their breasts to allow other family members to share in the feedings and give them a break. Since many triplets or more start off as premies, it's sometimes necessary to supplement breast milk until the babies' weight gains are sufficient. Supplementing is discussed in chapter 6. With three or four babies, it's also important to keep track of who nurses when, for how long, and how many wet diapers and bowel movements each infant has per day. (See chapter 6.)

COMMON PROBLEMS

There are usually a few kinks to work out before breastfeeding becomes a natural-born instinct for both you and baby. Here are some of the more common setbacks new mothers run into.

Feeding a Sleepy Baby

After delivery, it usually takes a newborn about twenty to thirty minutes of looking around before she's interested in feeding. On the first feeding, it's recommended to feed for about thirty minutes while the baby's alert. This helps get you both off to a good start. Then, if the baby has not had any medications, she'll fall into a deep sleep and then wake up regularly at least every two to three hours to feed.

Unless the baby's feeding every two to three hours at first, your body will not be able to establish the right amount of milk. In order to do this, your newborn needs to nurse at least eight to twelve times in a twenty-four-hour period. Each feeding should consist of active nursing for at least ten to fifteen minutes at each breast so the baby can obtain the hindmilk and stimulate the production of more milk. You should hear the baby swallowing after every one or two sucks once your milk letdown has occurred. Swallows become less frequent later in the feeding.

Babies usually grow out of their sleepiness in the first couple of weeks of life. In the meantime, here are some suggestions for feeding sleepy babies.

Waking the Baby

There is a solution to feeding a sleepy baby: Wake up the baby to feed, and if need be, wake up the baby during suckling if he keeps falling asleep at the breast.

Prior to waking the baby, try to determine whether he's in a deep or light sleep. In a lighter sleep state, the baby's eyes are moving under the eyelids, the lips make sucking movements, and the body is stirring. It's easier to rouse the baby from a lighter sleep. Touching the baby gently will usually wake him from a lighter sleep.

Cooling off helps rouse a baby from a deeper sleep. Do this by loosening or removing blankets or unwrapping the baby down to the diaper if the room is warm. A baby is the right temperature if the head is warm and the hands cool. Warm hands or a sweaty neck means the baby is too hot.

If this doesn't work, try to elicit some reflexes by supporting the baby's head while the upper body rests along your forearms. The baby's buttocks will rest on your abdomen if you're sitting up or on your chest if you're lying down. Then slowly bring your forearms forward, until the baby's head almost touches you, and then quickly move the baby away again. You'll probably need to repeat this a few times for the baby to open his eyes. As soon as he does, try to get him to look at you and follow your eyes while you move your head from side to side. Talk, sing, or coo while you do this. ("Hello . . . look who's awake? Are you awake? Hello there!") Once you catch the baby's attention, this is the time to call on your latch-on technique and begin to breastfeed.

Other waking techniques include using your fingertips to gently "walk" up the sides of the baby's spine from the buttocks to the base of the skull; circling the outside of the baby's lips a few times with your index finger; stroking the bottom of the baby's feet; and giving the baby a body massage.

Keeping the Baby Alert during Feeding

Sleepy babies tend to fall asleep as soon as they begin feeding. If your baby does this after only a few minutes of nursing, undress the baby down to the diaper to cool her off and keep her more alert. You can also switch breasts *before the breast is empty*. Keep moving the baby back and forth from one breast to the other until both breasts are empty. This provides more milk with less effort for the baby.

If your breasts are not completely empty by the end of the feeding, express/pump your milk to keep up your supply. Experts suggest that you also talk to your baby while she nurses, or play cheerful, lively music. Here are some other ways to keep the baby alert during nursing:

- Position the baby's head higher than her body.
- Gently massage the baby's crown in a circular motion.
- Stroke the baby's spine, tugging at your breast (if there's a good, strong latch), or stretch the corners of the baby's mouth by quickly pushing outward in opposite directions with your thumb and forefinger.
- Keep the room cooler. You can always cover the baby by blanket if necessary. Babies will fall asleep if they're too warm.
- Between sides, change the baby's diaper or burp the baby in a sitting-up position.
- Dim the lights during nursing. Bright lights may make the baby close her eyes.
- Manipulate baby's arms and legs in a gentle pat-a-cake game.

ஜ Wipe the baby's forehead and cheeks with a cool, damp cloth.

ஜ Express milk onto the baby's lips.

Why Is My Baby So Sleepy?

There are a number of reasons. First, have the baby's health checked out to rule out an underlying medical condition. Beyond that, if you experienced a difficult labor and delivery and certain drugs were given to you for pain relief, these drugs can make the baby overly sleepy and even interfere with his ability to suckle.

If the baby has received any supplements, such as water, formula, juice, or cereal, his appetite will be satisfied, which will make him lose interest in breastfeeding. That's why it's so important NOT to supplement the baby unless there's a good medical reason. The more full the baby is, the more sleepy he becomes. (We get sleepy too after a full meal.) By the way, any missed feedings should be replaced by an expressing/pumping session.

Finally, some babies sleep to avoid distractions, such as noise or lights. If this seems to describe your baby, try to nurse in a quiet, dark room, and experiment with different "white noise" tapes, such as waves and so on.

How Often Should I Wake the Baby at Night to Feed?

If you're having trouble establishing a milk supply, or if your baby is sleepy, wake the baby if she is still sleeping four hours after the last feeding started. For an accurate timing, count the interval from the *start* of each feeding to the start of the next. If the baby's last feeding began at 10:30 P.M., for example, and she finished both breasts by 11:00 P.M., the next feeding should begin at 2:30 A.M., not 3:00 A.M. (If your baby is breastfeeding well and thriving, don't wake her up; she'll wake you!)

My Baby Wasn't Sleepy until My Milk Came In! What's Going On?

Sometimes babies will fall asleep after milk letdown occurs because they're overwhelmed by the tremendous increase in milk compared with the colostrum. More swallowing action is needed to get the milk, and sometimes babies are taken aback by the extra effort. The baby needs to get used to the "new rules" of suckling and swallowing more frequently. The only way to do this is to keep breastfeeding and try to keep the baby alert while feeding, using the techniques discussed above. If the baby can't keep up, see an LC or the baby's doctor to try to determine how to solve the problem. Keep up your milk supply by pumping until the problem is resolved. Also see chapter 6, if you need to find an alternate way to feed the baby.

When Baby Pulls Away from the Breast

This is a frustrating problem for mother and baby alike, but there is usually a logical explanation for the behavior.

Babies may pull away because they either don't like the position they're being held in, or they're sensitive to where the mother's fingers are placed on their bodies.

For instance, when someone taps you on the shoulder, your immediate instinct is to turn around. It's the same thing with many babies. As soon as they feel a finger on one side of their face, they may also immediately turn around. Therefore, any position where you're touching the baby's face or head can produce a "What *is* that?" reflex. The solution: Stop doing it. If you must touch the baby's face or head, do it in a firm, constant way so you're not distracting the baby.

Your hand should be at the shoulders and base of the baby's head, providing support for the head, neck, and shoulders, with your fingertips behind and below the level of the baby's ears.

Sometimes babies pull away from the breast because your milk letdown is way too forceful. This is discussed next.

When Your Cup Runneth Over (Overactive Letdown)

An overactive letdown can be just as problematic as a poor letdown or a deficient milk supply. This is sometimes called forceful milk-ejection reflex (letdown). Your baby may choke and sputter and even pull away to let the heaviest part of the flow go by before latching on again.

As soon as you feel the letdown reflex, detach the baby from the breast when the milk starts to flow. Use a towel, glass, or bottle to catch the overflow. Put the baby on the breast when the flow subsides.

Also, position the baby in an "uphill" position, with his neck and throat higher than the nipple. This means that if you're in the football hold, lean back; in the cradle hold, prop the baby in your lap on two pillows and lean back in a rocking chair or recliner; and when lying down, place a folded towel under the baby so that he looks down toward the breast.

For a completely different position, nurse in the Australia position, where the baby lies on top of you while you lie flat on your back and support the baby's forehead with your hand. The excess milk will trickle out the sides of the baby's mouth and onto a diaper or towel.

A different problem may arise if you have an overabundant milk supply, which simply means that you're generally making too much breast milk—more than the baby needs. This is discussed in chapter 8 (page 215) because it is often the cause of a fussy, gassy baby.

When You're Leaking

It's very common to begin leaking milk out of one breast when you breast-feed from the other. As we've said, the sight, sound, or even thought of your baby can trigger milk letdown, and hence leaking, if there is no mouth at the end of the nipple.

In general, leaking tends to happen during the first few weeks of breast-feeding and tapers off as you and your baby establish the right milk supply. But some women will experience leaking for months—and that, too, is perfectly normal. Sometimes leaking may be a sign that your breasts are overly full. In this case, rather than holding back the milk it's best to express it. Leaking may also be a sign that you have an overabundant milk supply.

Turning Off the Tap

To stop your milk flow, apply gentle pressure directly on the nipples when leaking occurs. You can also fold your arms firmly across your chest; put the heels of your hands directly on your nipples; or put your hands under your chin and press against your breasts with your forearms.

Nursing pads, of course, come in handy, but make sure you use nursing pads made from natural fibers and without plastic in them, which can cause bacteria buildup. Wear clothing, too, that will camouflage wetness, such as print blouses, or have an extra jacket or sweater ready to cover up the stains.

When Your Letdown Reflex Isn't Working!

As discussed on page 98, the letdown reflex can take some time to kick in. Letdown can also be delayed if you're under stress—such as *worrying* about your letdown. (This is similar to worrying that you might be pregnant, which delays your period even more!) Finally, if your baby isn't latched on properly, your letdown may not be stimulated.

If your latch and positioning are correct and letdown is still not occurring, consult your doctor or an LC. As a last resort, there's a wonderful little product on the market in the form of an oxytocin nasal spray. This spray exactly duplicates the hormone oxytocin, which is normally stimulated by your baby's suckling. Your doctor can prescribe it to you, but you must use it *sparingly*. If your doctor suggests that you take the oxytocin spray at the beginning of each feeding for the first day or so, this is still too much. One spritz should do it. Otherwise, you run the risk of becoming conditioned to the stuff.

In the worst-case scenario, colostrum may not be coming out either. The solution is to supplement by feeding tube at the breast (see chapter 6) so the baby can still stimulate your breasts. When letdown is better established, you then simply switch to normal breastfeeding.

The Arching Baby

This is another frustrating problem, where the baby arches her head and body away from the breast and screams every time you start to nurse. In some cases, arching babies even roll away from the breast.

One common reason for this is that the breast isn't satisfying the baby's hunger. The baby's behavior is telling you: "Look—this isn't working for me!" The source of this problem is usually either a bad latch, having the breast forced on the baby, or even a weak suck. But an overactive letdown (see above) or colic (see chapter 8) can cause arching too. In the case of a bad latch, unless it's corrected, the hindmilk will not be available to satisfy the baby's hunger.

If arching is a problem, first have the baby's health evaluated to rule out an underlying medical condition. Then see an LC to make sure that your position and latch are correct. Sometimes just nursing in a different position will resolve things. A variety of different nursing positions can prevent the arch and support the baby. Express your milk via pump to keep up your milk supply until the problem is solved.

How to Feed an Arching Baby

These babies need some calming before nursing. You can do this by massage or by holding the baby firmly. Sometimes after a few arches the baby may just settle down to nurse.

Try a modified version of the football hold to nurse the baby. Position the baby's buttocks against a hard surface with legs pointing upward so the feet do not touch anything (this may trigger an arch). Hold the baby's head so the chin almost touches the chest, which helps the tongue move correctly. Elevate your leg so that your thigh can support the arm holding the baby. A pillow or folded blanket can also help support your hand and forearm.

Arching babies can also nurse well in the cradle position if they're held firmly in a cloth nursing sling. The sling helps prevent your arms and shoulders from getting tired.

When You're Exhausted

Many women find it difficult to adjust to the lack of sleep that comes with caring for a newborn (it's worse with bottle-feeding, by the way). The best advice is: When in Rome, do as the Romans do—or in this case, as the baby does. Sleep when the baby sleeps; eat when the baby eats. Some women find carrying the baby in a sling between feedings helpful; they don't have to run back and forth to check on the baby, and can even do some simple chores around the house or make phone calls.

When Your Baby Isn't Thriving

This is an extremely common concern for all parents, whether they're breastfeeding or not. That's why it's important to read chapter 6, "When to Supplement," which discusses what to look for in babies who are thriving and the symptoms of babies who require medical attention or supplements. Warning signs to watch for:

- Fewer than 6 (disposable) or 8 (cloth) soaked diapers in 24 hours (see chapter 6).

- Persistent diarrhea (see chapters 6 and 8).

- Jaundice (see chapter 8).

- Fever (can mean an infection or illness: see chapter 8).

- Persistent weight loss (see chapter 6).

- Persistent crying (see chapter 8).

When you notice any of these things, immediately contact your baby's doctor.

Should You Sleep with Your Baby?

Well, yes—according to new findings. Sharing your bed with your infant is called "bedsharing" in clinical circles. Studies show that bedsharing infants breastfeed approximately three times longer during the night than infants who routinely slept separately, which means that it may help protect against sudden infant death syndrome (SIDS). Of course, the more you breastfeed, the less likely you are to resume ovulation (see chapter 10), which will help with child spacing and protection against ovarian cancer. Why do bedsharing babies breastfeed more often? Apparently, they can smell their mother's breast milk, making them turn toward the mother. A mother will also sense when her infant is waking up and is more apt to breastfeed.

When You Receive Free Formula

Formula companies have a way of finding you when you deliver. Sales representatives may routinely call hospitals to get a list of new maternity patients. Then, in an attempt to get your business, they'll send you free cases of formula, and may even send you gift baskets with a variety of baby products, such as baby foods, cereals, pacifiers, toys, and so on. Hospitals are sent gift boxes of free samples too, and encouraged to send them home with mother and baby.

Many women have confessed to me that these samples look mighty tempting when breastfeeding isn't going that well. But please keep in mind that every time you give your baby a bottle of formula instead of your breast, your breasts will make less milk. As you give more bottles, your milk supply keeps dropping until you stop breastfeeding altogether. Then you have to *buy* formula, and the company has got you where they want you.

Formula companies don't give you these samples because they like you; they give you samples because they know it will help them to make a profit.

If you're like me, you'll find it difficult to just throw out all that free formula. So don't. You can donate it to women's shelters, food banks, or use it in your baking (as suggested in chapter 2) as a substitute for condensed milk. If you know of other mothers who are formula feeding, give *them* the formula. (Cats will drink the cow's-milk-based formulas too.)

ʕ๑

Clearly, the first week of breastfeeding can be overwhelming for the novice, but if expressing milk can be mastered, your milk supply will thrive, and engorgement will be avoided. Self-expression is such a central issue to good breastfeeding management that I've devoted the entire next chapter to the subject.

Figure 4-3

EVERY STEP COUNTS! HOW DOES YOUR NEIGHBORHOOD HOSPITAL/HEALTH FACILITY MEASURE UP? IS IT BABY-FRIENDLY?

Why should you act now? Taking the time to complete this evaluation and sharing it with the hospital administrators, health workers, and your friends can help improve the services in your community. You may wish to build on this questionnaire and link it with other activities to adapt to any special circumstances.

How can you make a difference?

1. Fill out this Baby-Friendly Hospital Initiative Survey.
2. All "Yes" responses are worth one point. Question 9 has different point values.
3. Add up all the points and write the total in the box provided.
4. Use this checklist when selecting maternity services and let hospital administrators know how their hospital compares to the global standard defined in the WHO/UNICEF Joint Statement.

	Yes	No	?
1. Before my baby was born, I was told why and how to breastfeed.	___	___	___
2. The staff were knowledgeable and supportive of breastfeeding.	___	___	___
3. I was shown how to breastfeed my baby.	___	___	___
4. I was encouraged and helped to breastfeed without the use of any other foods or liquids for my baby.	___	___	___
5. My breasts were examined before and after my baby's birth.	___	___	___
6. I was instructed to breastfeed whenever my baby wanted to suck or cried.	___	___	___
7. At birth, my baby's weight was recorded on a growth chart, which was given to me.	___	___	___
8. My baby and I had skin-to-skin contact immediately following the birth.	___	___	___
9. I offered my baby the breast for the first time within: ___ 30 min. (2 pts) ___ 1 hour (1 pt) ___ more than 1 hour (0 pt)			
10. My baby was not given food or drink by the staff.	___	___	___
11. My baby and I were not separated at any time during our hospital stay.	___	___	___
12. My baby was not given any rubber nipples or pacifiers by the staff.	___	___	___
13. I was not given any formula, breast-milk substitutes, bottles, or rubber nipples when I left the hospital.	___	___	___
14. I was told when my baby would need to be examined and weighed and how to schedule an appointment for her/him.	___	___	___

Figure 4-3 continued

	Yes	No	?
15. I was told how to contact a breastfeeding mother's support group when I was discharged from care.	___	___	___
16. The hospital has a written breastfeeding policy that reflects the WHO/UNICEF "10 Steps" and International Code.	___	___	___
17. Overall, I believe my breastfeeding experience was improved by this facility.	___	___	___

Remember: To total the score, add all the points and compare to the chart below. Send this form to the hospital administrator. You may wish to include a personal note. Keep a record of this form for yourself and your community/county committee.

Total Score _____

How does your community hospital measure up?

18–19 Congratulations! Your facility is doing a wonderful job in protecting, supporting, and promoting breastfeeding.

15–18 Keep up the good work! You are effectively helping breastfeeding mothers and babies. Find out how you can be even more helpful by contacting one of the sponsoring organizations.

12–15 Your facility could do much more to assist breastfeeding. The sponsoring organizations have technical assistance available for suggestions on how to implement the Ten Steps.

  0–12 Breastfeeding mothers and babies are having a difficult time at your facility. Find out why these issues are important. Begin to make changes that will increase your patients' satisfaction and improve infant health.

Reprinted with permission of the World Alliance for Breastfeeding Action (WABA).

chapter 5

ℰXPRESSING 𝒴OURSELF

ave you ever cooked dinner for a dozen guests? If you have, you know how important timing your meal is. The best dinner-party hosts need to juggle a variety of cooking tasks, keeping some foods warm without burning or drying them out while keeping other, cold foods crisp and fresh. Add in the garlic bread, the fruit tray, the ice, chilling the wine, and broiling various appetizers, and you have a delicate food-management story. And what about guests who are late? Guests who are vegetarians? Guests who have various food allergies? Weather problems that may delay your dinner party? All these come with the territory of everyday party hosting that many of us have dealt with. As a result, most of us have tricks regarding food preparation, such as cooking dishes in advance; using tin foil to keep food from drying out or burning; employing the microwave to speed up cooking times; and so on. But we've *learned* all of these tricks—we weren't born with the knowledge.

Well, expressing/pumping your breast milk actually works on the same principle as meal preparation but—it's a lot easier. Like any cook, you must provide your baby with enough fresh food to keep him satisfied. It's simple, really. When you make too much food, you need to freeze the extra food, and when you don't have enough food on the table, you need to make more.

Expressing/pumping your own milk is so crucial for good breast-feeding management that this entire chapter is devoted to the subject. As mentioned before, many women will need to express/pump their milk at some point during breastfeeding, while others will need to express/pump several times a day. The consequences of not emptying your breasts frequently can lead to a dwindling milk supply and even engorgement from an overabundant milk supply. So it's important to know how to empty your breasts yourself, for those times when your baby cannot.

Expressing/pumping your own milk will also build up a "reserve stash," which can be given to your baby anytime a supplement is needed. Supplements, as you'll see in chapter 6, do *not* necessarily mean formula or sugar water. Your own milk is the best supplement there is. For women who want to resume breastfeeding after they've already weaned, or who have given up too early in the game, expressing/pumping their milk can help to *reestablish* their milk supply, in what is known as relactation. Meanwhile, some women who have never breastfed or even experienced pregnancy may be able to induce lactation through pumping milk (more effective than hand expressing in this case). Both relactation and induced lactation are discussed at the end of this chapter.

Before you read on, however, review the section in chapter 3 entitled A Consumer's Guide to Breast Pumps. (I specifically put that section in chapter 3 because I think all women who plan to breastfeed should look into breast pumps before they deliver, so that if they end up needing one they'll know which pump to get.) While information on the Marmet technique of hand expression is provided in figure 5-1, on the following page, many women find it easier to learn the technique when *shown* how do it in person or by video. Any La Leche League leader (see the appendix) or a woman skilled in hand expressing can help you get the hang of it. A doctor, nurse, midwife, or LC can also demonstrate the technique.

WHO, WHAT, WHEN, WHERE, AND WHY

The basics of milk expressing/pumping come down to the five Ws: who should express milk and why; when to express milk and where; and finally, what to use to get the job done.

Who Should Express/Pump Herself?

In the same way that no two pregnancies—even for the same woman—are alike, no two breastfeeding experiences are alike. Each baby will develop a particular feeding schedule, while each woman will have certain adjustments to make based on her physique, her baby's health and physique, her

Figure 5-1
MARMET TECHNIQUE OF MANUAL EXPRESSION OF BREAST MILK

Expressing the Milk
Draining the Milk Reservoirs

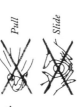

1. *Position* the thumb and first two fingers about 1" to 1½" (2.5 cm to 4 cm) behind the nipple.
   - Use this measurement, which is not necessarily the outer edge of the areola, as a guide. The areola varies in size from one woman to another.
   - Place the thumb pad above the nipple and the finger pads below the nipple forming the letter "C" with the hand, as shown.
   - Note that the fingers are positioned so that the milk reservoirs lie beneath them.
   - Avoid cupping the breast.

2. *Push* straight into the chest wall.
   - Avoid spreading the fingers apart.
   - For large breasts, first lift and then push into the chest wall.

Push into chest wall

3. *Roll* thumb and fingers forward as if making thumb and fingerprints at the same time.
   - The rolling motion of the thumb and fingers compresses and empties the milk reservoirs with-out hurting sensitive breast tissue.
   - Note the moving position of the thumbnail and fingernails in the illustration.

Roll

Finish roll

4. *Repeat rhythmically* to drain the reservoirs.
   - Position, push, roll; position, push, roll . . .

5. *Rotate* the thumb and finger position to milk the other reservoirs. Use both hands on each breast. These pictures show hand positions on the right breast.

Right hand *Left hand*

Avoid These Motions

Avoid squeezing the breast. This can cause bruising.

Squeeze

Avoid pulling out the nipple and breast. This can cause tissue damage.

Pull

Avoid sliding on the breast. This can cause skin burns.

Slide

Assisting the Milk Ejection Reflex
Stimulating the Flow of Milk

Massage

1. *Massage* the milk-producing cells and ducts.
   - Start at the top of the breast. Press firmly into the chest wall. Move fingers in a circular motion on one spot on the skin.
   - After a few seconds, move the fingers to the next area on the breast.
   - Spiral around the breast toward the areola using this massage.
   - The motion is similar to that used in a breast examination.

2. *Stroke* the breast area from the top of the breast to the nipple with a light, ticklelike stroke.
   - Continue this stroking motion from the chest wall to the nipple around the whole breast.
   - This will help with relaxation and will help stimulate the milk ejection reflex.

Stroke

3. *Shake* the breast while leaning forward so that gravity will help the milk eject.

Shake

Manual Expression of Breastmilk—Marmet Technique. Copyright 1978, revised 1979, 1981 and 1988 Chele Marmet. Used with permission of Chele Marmet and The Lactation Institute, 16430 Ventura Blvd., Ste. 303, Encino, CA 91436, USA.

home and work environments, and the level of breastfeeding support and information she's receiving.

One or more of the following situations may require women to express/pump their milk:

- *Breastfeeding isn't going well.* You and your baby are having some scheduling problems. Expressing/pumping your milk will keep up your milk supply until you and the baby get it right.

- *Baby isn't thriving.* Whether your baby is a premie or has a minor or major health problem, don't allow the baby to subsist on "artificial food." There's nothing like your home-cooked meals to get your baby's health back. Pumping will allow for breast milk to be given to a baby who's not well enough to breastfeed or needs extra nourishment. (See chapter 6 for more details on when and who to supplement, and the variety of supplementation methods available.)

- *You're going back to work.* Think of expressing/pumping your milk as a trip to the grocery store. You may not have time to do it, but you have to *make* the time in order to bring home fresh food for your family to eat. (At least you don't have to worry about parking— something you *would* need to think about if you had to go the store to buy formula!) Expressing/pumping your milk on the job can be done even in the most ultraconservative workplace. I'll tell you how in chapter 9.

- *You are nursing more than one baby.* The more children a family has, the more food that family needs to make during mealtime. Expressing/pumping your milk after feedings will build up your milk supply so you can feed more than one mouth at a time. Remember, it's supply and demand. The more demand, the more supply!

- *Whenever a nursing is missed.* Skipped nursings will bring on engorgement and cause your milk supply to dwindle. *Every time your baby skips a nursing (for whatever reason), replace it with an expressing/pumping session.* This will keep your feeding schedule on track, keep your milk supply up, and prevent engorgement.

- *You don't have enough milk.* This is often the case if your breasts are not emptied effectively or often enough. Expressing/pumping your milk after feedings will stimulate the whole process. In a single-baby situation, poor milk supply is often the result of poor latching and positioning. In this case, breastfeed as much and for as long as the baby wants, and make sure your technique isn't the problem. If your technique is okay, begin to express/pump your milk after feedings. This will signal your brain to send down more milk, because it will think that the breast pump is your baby. (See chapter 4, page 98, for more details on poor letdown.) If there's no milk to express after nursing, pumping/expressing will help slightly, but you may need a lactagogue. But if there is no milk after nursing and your baby is thriving, you're fine. Finally, if there is milk left to pump after a feeding and your baby is not thriving, this indicates a problem with the latch (see chapter 4) or the baby's health (see chapters 6 and 8).

જ *You have too much milk.* When your milk supply is overabundant, you'll need to express your breasts, not to empty them but just until you're comfortable. This will prevent engorgement. See chapter 8 for more details on too much breast milk, and chapter 4 for details on an overactive letdown (a different problem).

જ *You need to temporarily stop breastfeeding.* In certain circumstances, you may need to stop breastfeeding and then resume it later on. This would be the case if you needed to be separated from your baby for any reason, be it hospitalization (you may be able to stay with your baby), undergoing a therapy that is unsafe during breastfeeding (you can ask for alternative medications safe for breastfeeding), or if you needed to travel out of town for business or pleasure (see if you can take the baby with you). If you're stuck and must be separated, then expressing/pumping your milk to mimic the feeding schedule your baby had will keep your milk supply up for when you're able to breastfeed again.

When to Express/Pump Yourself

The answer largely depends on why you're expressing/pumping.

If your baby isn't breastfeeding at all due to illness or hospitalization, you'll need to regularly express your milk to mimic a normal breastfeeding schedule, which is roughly every two to three hours, or ten to twelve times every twenty-four hours, with a good, full-size electric pump. If your baby is very young, your purpose is to build up a milk supply. Otherwise, every three hours by day and once at night with the electric pump should do the trick and keep up a milk supply for when your baby is ready to breastfeed.

It's also normal for your milk supply to fluctuate with the baby's condition. As discussed in chapter 4, stress can inhibit adequate milk letdown; what could be more stressful than having a baby in the hospital? If your milk supply has dwindled slightly, increase the number of times you pump. If your milk supply is still inadequate, see your doctor about lactagogues.

If you're breastfeeding *sometimes* but are experiencing problems with latching, positioning, physical challenges, or any other obstacle discussed in chapter 4, express/pump your milk at the following times:

- Whenever the baby hasn't emptied your breasts completely.
- Whenever you've skipped a nursing—particularly if you're temporarily separated from your baby.
- Whenever your breasts are overfull with milk.

At the same time, see your doctor or LC to try to correct your breastfeeding problem, whatever it may be.

If you're going back to work and have your baby in a day-care center or under the supervision of a nanny, express/pump your breasts approximately when you would normally feed your baby if you *were* at home. That milk can be kept in the fridge (storage issues are discussed further on), brought home, and fed to your baby the next day. For nighttime feedings, carry on as usual and breastfeed directly. In essence, nothing has changed in terms of your schedule—you're just delivering your food later. (See chapter 9 for more details.)

HOW TO MILK IT FOR ALL IT'S WORTH

As you probably already know, the more you milk, the more you get. Unless the breasts are regularly emptied, milk production will back up and back*fire*! You'll get engorged, and then your milk supply will dwindle. So in order to milk your breasts for all they're worth, if your baby can't do it, then either hand-express (see figure 5-1) or do it with an electric, double-setup breast pump. (See chapter 3, A Consumer's Guide to Breast Pumps, page 77, for more details.)

If you're trying your hand at manual expressing, it may take a week or two to build up enough strength in your hand muscles. Squeezing a rubber ball or other hand exerciser will help. With a big rental electric pump with a double setup, however, you can pump both breasts at once and save time. Double pumping also most effectively stimulates the breasts to produce more milk—particularly if you have more than one baby. If you haven't yet read the breast pump section in chapter 3, *go back and do it now*. Once you've chosen the pump product that's right for you, read on.

Getting Pumped Up

Chapter 3 discusses a variety of breast pump products on the market. To briefly recap, the best breast pump you can rent or buy is electric with an automatic cycle for the suction pressure, to imitate a baby's suckling cycle. *Avoid pumps that require you to turn the suction on and off yourself* (by sliding your thumb off and on a hole in the suction system).

Big electric pumps with a double setup are the most effective for breast emptying. At roughly three dollars a day (less than a day's worth of formula) to rent, this is a particularly good deal if you have to pump often.

Finally, as discussed in chapter 3, a manual pump is convenient and effective if you are traveling and cannot take your big electric pump along.

How Do I Get Started?

Start with clean hands to avoid transferring bacteria. Next, begin to trigger your letdown; unless letdown occurs, pumping will not be effective. Gently massage your breasts and try to think about your baby, imagining, perhaps, the feeling of the baby nursing. Looking at baby pictures, smelling some of your baby's clothes, or watching videotapes of the baby may help. (This can all be done while you're pumping; you'll just pick up the pace when letdown occurs.) Also review the Letdown Foreplay section in chapter 4.

Or you can begin pumping once you feel your letdown occur. If you're pumping only one side at a time, pump the fullest side first. Set your electric pump to the gentlest setting and work to the strongest if necessary. Too strong a setting can damage sensitive breast tissue.

At first, your milk will drip; then, after letdown, it will spray into the container (which often comes with the pump). When you begin to see drips again instead of sprays, you can stop pumping. If you're pumping one side at a time, do side one until it drips; do side two until it drips; then return to side one to get the last little bit; and same again to side two.

The time it takes you to pump your breasts should about equal the time it takes for your baby to empty your breasts. The exception to this rule is when you're pumping both breasts at once.

The amount of milk you can pump in any one sitting largely depends on how long it's been since you last breastfed or expressed, how efficient you are at expressing/pumping (which is why manual expressing rarely gets the job done), how comfortable you are in your pumping "surroundings," the time of day, and your general milk supply. As discussed in chapter 4, stress can also inhibit letdown if you're in an uncomfortable setting or are not adept at using your pump.

If you're worried whether you're pumping as much milk as you should be, keep in mind that the baby's suckling will always be more efficient than even the best breast pump.

A myth is currently circulating regarding increasing your fluid intake to increase your chances of expressing/pumping more milk. More fluids will not mean more milk. As discussed in chapter 2, just drink when you're thirsty. The only things that will increase your milk supply are medication, expressing/pumping, or your baby's suckling.

Following Instructions

In addition to triggering your milk letdown prior to pumping, it's important to *read the instructions that came with your breast pump!* Some other pumping tips:

- ✍ Select a nipple adapter that's the right size. Size your nipple in its "at ease" position, and center it in the opening, with the flange just surrounding the nipple but not touching or rubbing against it.

- ✍ Moisten your breast just before pumping to improve the suction or the nipple adapter.

✍ Interrupt your pumping a few times to massage your breasts. This will help to stimulate more letdowns when you resume pumping.

✍ Switch breasts frequently. When you notice that your milk flow begins to dwindle, switch breasts instead of waiting for the bitter end. Pumping tends to work better if you give each breast short breaks.

When pumping is uncomfortable or painful, something's *wrong*. Double-check the instructions to make sure you're using the pump correctly. Sometimes all that's necessary is setting the pump pressure to a lower strength or trying a larger-size pump flange. When you resume pumping, begin on the side that's least sore first, and then pump the sore breast just enough to prevent engorgement instead of emptying it completely. If soreness persists, see if pumping more frequently for shorter periods of time helps. If all else fails, you may need to switch to a different kind of pump. (See chapter 3.)

The Best Time and Place

If you're pumping to build up a milk supply or to relieve breasts that haven't been properly emptied by the baby's suckling, pump after you have nursed. Choose the same nursing each day to build up a regular schedule. If you're pumping because you're separated from your baby or your baby has skipped a feeding, replace any missed nursing with a pumping session. At night, pumping once is sufficient.

If you're pumping because you're working, for example, pumping in the early morning may work best, when you're well rested. You'll be able to express more milk in a shorter period of time in the morning than at night, when you're tired and the baby is fussier.

Another option is to express a little milk several times a day instead of having a few longer sessions.

It's also possible to pump one breast while your baby suckles on the other, using a trigger handle pump or manually expressing. This has the advantage of the baby stimulating your milk letdown. This setup may occur where you're pumping to increase your milk supply. In this case, you can even feed your baby shortly after pumping. The suckling will just trigger more milk.

As for the best pumping zones: Anywhere you're comfortable pumping is a good place. If you're at work, you may need to get creative, but there are ways. (See chapter 9 for more details.) With a portable pump (see chapter 3), locations vary from private offices (in some workplaces) to public washrooms, fitting rooms in retail stores, and discreet places in malls or parks. Many women prefer to pump in washrooms where they can lean over a sink, which prevents dripping milk on clothing.

Make It a Ritual

When you're able to pump in the comfort of your own home, design your own "prepumping ritual" to get you in the right mood. This can include any activities that help to trigger milk letdown, such as watching baby videos or sitting in a comfortable chair and relaxing. Include some physical letdown triggers too, such as applying heat to your breast (a warm compress or heating pad), taking a bath or shower, massaging the breasts, stimulating your nipples, and so on.

If you're separated from your baby and are trying to pump in a hotel room, for example, call home before you pump to get yourself thinking about the baby. Once you get the hang of it, all you'll have to do is think about your baby and the milk will flow.

Washing Your Equipment

After you've pumped, wash your hands in hot, soapy water and towel-dry. This will ensure that your pump is kept as sterile as possible during handling.

Any part of the pump that comes into contact with the breast or milk should be washed in hot, soapy water and then rinsed well. Bacteria tend to accumulate if dried particles of milk are left in the breast shield, tubing, or collection bottle. It's usually not necessary to sterilize these parts, unless you're feeding the milk to a very sick or weak baby. To do this, stick the pump parts on the top rack of the dishwasher and run them through a sanicycle after you've handwashed them. If you don't have a dishwasher, put the equipment in a big soup cauldron, fill it with water and a tablespoon of white vinegar, and boil it for a full five minutes. Then use sterile tongs to lift out the pump parts, and set them to cool on a dry counter or fresh cloth. When everything's dry, assemble the equipment and put it in a clean, airtight bag or container until you need to use it again.

STORING AND SERVING HUMAN MILK

There is a milk storage bag product for this, specifically designed for freezing and storing human milk. The most popular brand, Mother's Milk Freezing Bags, can be purchased through La Leche League International (see the appendix). These bags are superior for storing human milk because they're two-ply, coated with polyethylene, and lined with nylon, so the fat cells in human milk will not adhere to the bag and will get into the baby. They're also self-sealing, presterilized, and have areas for labeling your "freshness" date.

While you can also use disposable bottle liners to freeze your milk, they're not as durable and can cause all kinds of problems. First, it's almost impossible to remove air from these liners without spilling milk all over the place. Second, you may find that the seams of these liners burst during freezing or leak during thawing.

Finally, if you're using bottle liners for a hospitalized baby, it can become contaminated when hospital staff attempt to remove the milk.

If you don't have any milk storage bags, the following make good milk containers:

- Sterile bottles (leave about an inch at the top for expansion when freezing).

- Tupperware that's been run through the sani-cycle of your dishwasher.

- Ice-cube trays run through the sani-cycle; frozen cubes can later be transferred into another container.

If you want to use disposable bottle liners to freeze your milk, here are the rules:

1. Double-bag it.

2. Squeeze out the air at the top.

3. Roll down the bag to about one inch above the milk.

4. Close the bag and seal it tightly.

5. Place the sealed bag upright in a heavy plastic container with a lid, and seal the lid before putting it in the freezer.

6. *Never use Baggies or household-use plastic bags!* They break.

If your baby is ill or premature, let the hospital staff know about which storage container you plan to use, and ask if there are any special storage requirements you need to adhere to. You may also want to check with the neonatal staff about the amount of milk to store in each container.

A Word about Glass

When it comes to storing milk, plastic or glass makes no difference if your baby is healthy and thriving. But since valuable white blood cells in fresh milk stored in glass tend to cling to the glass and never get inside the baby, this might have an effect on an ill or premature infant. If you're freezing the milk anyway, there's no way to preserve these white blood cells; they'll die in either plastic or glass.

Freezing and Refrigeration

The old storage rules for breast milk maintain that its shelf life in the refrigerator did not extend beyond forty-eight hours. Research from a 1987 study, however, found that human milk has unique, bacteria-resistant properties that allow it to stay fresh longer, so it is now possible to refrigerate breast milk for up to five days before freezing it.

Mature breast milk (i.e., not colostrum) can be kept frozen for up to two weeks in a fridge-top freezer. In a separate-door freezer, it'll keep for up to three months (at the back rather than on the door), and in a big-chest freezer (at −18°C or lower), it'll keep for six months.

Lactation experts suggest that you freeze only about three to four ounces of milk at a time. This is about the quantity your baby would get in a feeding, and prevents you from wasting milk the baby doesn't drink. Moreover, it's easier to thaw smaller quantities of milk. To produce less wasted milk, freeze in two-ounce servings and just combine with other freezings to make a full serving.

The Recipe for Freezing

Use your "soup rules" here. Never freeze the milk immediately after pumping. Cool it down first in a fridge or small cooler with ice packs. Once the milk is cooled, it can be poured on top of previously frozen milk and put back in the freezer to freeze a new layer. Or you can start a new container. Don't pour warm milk on top of frozen milk, though, or you'll thaw the previously frozen milk.

Do I Have to Freeze It Right Away?

No; breast milk can be left out at room temperature for up to ten hours, as long as it's covered. Colostrum can be kept at room temperature for up to twenty-four hours before freezing; then follow the mature-milk freezing rules.

Milk can also be stored in the fridge for an additional forty-eight hours before it's frozen. Then it will keep in a connected freezer compartment for two weeks, as mentioned earlier, and at the back of a separate-door freezer for up to three months.

Label all your containers with the date that the contents were express/pumped, and count ahead to create your own freshness date based on the type of freezer you have. If several days' worth of milk are in one container, put the date of the earliest collection on the container. If the milk will be used in a day-care facility where more than one baby is in attendance, put the baby's name on the label too. If your baby is hospitalized, you'll need to put your own name, your baby's name, and the date you expressed the milk on the label. Always serve the earliest date first. Throw out any milk that is past its freshness date.

Thawing and Reheating

Many women are surprised to see how their milk, after it's been stored for a few days, separates into milk and cream. This is perfectly normal. Those of us who grew up drinking homogenized milk aren't accustomed to this sight. If your milk has separated, just shake the container before you feed it to your baby. Your milk may also turn shades of blue, yellow, or brown. This happens because of the foods you eat, which can color your milk.

Human milk shouldn't be "overcooked." That's why microwaves are not suitable for thawing breast milk. Some parts of the milk will be overheated, which could scald your baby, while certain infection-fighting properties of the milk will be destroyed when heated over 130°F.

The proper way to thaw milk is to place the frozen bag or bottle in a pot of warm tap water or to hold it under running warm tap water with the lid or twist tie above the water level. The breast milk should be shaken gently while you're thawing it.

Then take the milk and transfer it into one of the feeders discussed in chapter 6 (a variety of feeders are available that do not involve rubber nipples or bottle-feeding). Mission accomplished.

One last word: At the risk of sounding like your mother-in-law, if you're counting on a baby-sitter or nanny to feed your previously stored breast milk to your baby, do be sure to go over all the above rules regarding storage and thawing.

WHO IS A STORED MILK CUSTOMER?

It's good to know who your customer base comprises when it comes to expressed/pumped human milk. The following babies will benefit from expressed/pumped milk:

- Babies who have trouble getting the breast milk at the breast, such as those who are neurologically impaired, those with cardiac problems, some babies with Down syndrome, some premature babies, and some babies with a cleft palate (see Nursing a Cleft Palate in chapter 4). Chapter 6 discusses when it is appropriate to supplement, and chapter 8 discusses a variety of infant health problems.

- Any baby who isn't getting enough breast milk for any reason. Chapters 4, 6, 7, and 8 discuss a variety of situations that could cause malnourishment due to breastfeeding problems (poor latch and so on) or an underlying medical condition. In this case, expressed milk fed to the baby in one of the feeders discussed briefly below and in chapter 6 will get that baby's health back on track.

𝄢 A baby who isn't latching onto the breast properly or is "nipple confused" (see chapter 4).

𝄢 A baby whose mother is relactating (see the next section) and needs to be supplemented by a feeding tube at the breast.

How to Feed Expressed/Pumped Milk

If your baby is breastfeeding either regularly or occasionally and requires supplements, bottle-feeding will interfere with the baby's latch when she goes back to the breast. Any baby who can bottle-feed, however, can breastfeed so long as she is not nipple confused. Again, bottle-feeding is a problem only if your baby is also suckling at the breast.

RELACTATION TECHNIQUES

When a woman decides to resume breastfeeding (with either the same or another child) after she's weaned one child already, the process is called relactation. Relactation is also possible for a woman who has weaned her baby at birth. There is generally no statute of limitations for a woman who wants to relactate. Relactation is just as possible for a woman who weaned six years ago as it is for a woman who weaned six months ago. But the more recently you've been pregnant and have weaned, and the more abundant your milk supply was before weaning, the easier it will be to build up your milk supply now. (For women who have not weaned recently, the lactagogue domperidone may be a good idea.) In this case, regularly pumping your breasts will begin to trigger the milk production hormones and help you rebuild your milk supply.

If you've never been pregnant before but would like to breastfeed, there is a process known as *induced lactation*, discussed below. Induced lactation would be an alternative for an adopted baby, for example.

Relactation is not to be confused with *tandem nursing*, which is breastfeeding right through to another pregnancy, then continuing breastfeeding *during* that pregnancy, and then after the delivery of another child. (Tandem nursing is discussed more in chapter 10.)

Reasons to Relactate

Every woman will have different reasons to relactate. Here are some common ones:

- Changing your mind about weaning. If you've weaned but have reconsidered, you may want to relactate.
- Your baby is allergic or intolerant to regular milk or formula, and you need to return to breastfeeding for the baby's health.
- The baby has developed a serious medical condition and breast milk will help restore the baby's health faster.
- You're breastfeeding a relative or friend's baby because the natural mother cannot breastfeed (due to previous surgery, for example).
- You're breastfeeding an infant born prematurely or ill who was not supplemented with your own milk in the hospital.
- You're breastfeeding an adopted baby (but were pregnant before).

Assuming that your positioning and latch technique are correct and that your nipples are not inverted or flat, the success of your relactation effort will largely depend on how recently you weaned and how abundant your previous milk supply was. In addition, the effort also depends on the baby's age, response to the breast when it's reoffered, and familiarity with breastfeeding. A baby who breastfed for three months and is being rebreastfed at six months is more likely to respond with an "Oh, yeah—I remember this!" Meanwhile, a baby who has never breastfed and is being introduced to it for the first time at six months may have a difficult time latching onto the breast—particularly after feeding from a rubber nipple.

Finally, your spouse or family's support—or lack thereof—may also affect your relactation effort.

Getting Started—Again!

Once you've decided to relactate, it's a good idea to seek out other women who have also relactated. The resource list in the appendix offers organizations you can contact.

Ideally, having your baby suckle does the job more efficiently. But since it's not realistic to expect a baby to suckle for any significant length of time without actually getting milk, you'll need to supplement by feeding tube at the breast (see figure 6-1 on page 168). This allows the baby to get your expressed/pumped milk while also stimulating your breasts to make more milk.

Encourage comfort feedings, and put the baby onto your breast every few hours to try to establish a breastfeeding schedule. Rebuilding a milk supply also depends on how much milk you *want*. If you want to completely replace your baby's feedings with milk, it will take longer to rebuild the supply than if you just wanted enough milk for comfort or supplementary feedings. As always, the more often the baby breastfeeds, the more milk you'll make. Once you start menstruating again, you may also notice a slight decrease in your milk supply.

Milk Meds

Whether it's been a few months or over a year since you weaned, rebuilding a milk supply is highly variable. Consult your doctor about lactagogues, which will speed things up and allow a better breast milk supply to be established. As discussed earlier, lactagogues are medications (in pill form) that stimulate your prolactin levels and therefore your milk supply. These medications are NOT the same as oxytocin nasal sprays, discussed in the previous chapter, which are used to help with letdown.

Some women have reported success with certain herbs, but it's important to tell both your own doctor and your baby's doctor about any herbal medications you're using. Some can do more damage than good. Review table 2-7 in chapter 2.

WHEN YOU INDUCE LACTATION

Since the only time a woman would really need to induce lactation is for an adopted child, this process is also called "adoptive nursing." While the technique for inducing lactation is identical to that for relactation, I won't lie to you—it's difficult to accomplish when you've never been pregnant before, and even the most dedicated woman may find that her efforts to lactate produce no milk. In this case, the goal of breastfeeding is on establishing a satisfying nursing relationship, since the amount of milk a woman produces in this situation is highly variable.

Fortunately, lactation experts have compiled recommendations and suggestions over the years that can optimize the success of this process.

Give Yourself Some Time

Remember, it takes nine months of pregnancy before natural breastfeeding takes place, so give yourself some time to induce lactation. Begin to pump your breasts either two months before your baby arrives or as soon as you find out that you're getting your baby.

If you plan to adopt a child who hasn't been born yet, begin to pump your breasts as soon as the plans are confirmed (to the extent that they can be confirmed). That way, when the baby's born, if lactation is successful, you can begin breastfeeding ASAP. On the other hand, if you were unable to lactate, you will have had time to plan for an alternative (see chapters 2 and 6).

When the Baby Arrives but Your Milk Doesn't
If lactation is unsuccessful, don't hesitate to feed the baby at your breast using one of the supplementer feeders discussed in the next chapter. Look also into using a milk bank so you can feed donated breast milk to your baby instead of formula. Finally, you may want to ask your doctor about whether a lactagogue will help.

When You're Successful

If you've been successful in producing some breast milk, as soon as the baby arrives, try to replace your pumping session with your new baby's suckling. You may need to supplement with a feeding tube at the breast to ensure that the baby gets enough, but the suckling is a more efficient way to stimulate your milk supply. You may still need to continue expressing/pumping your milk until you and the baby get it right.

Keep in mind, though, that a baby's suckling cannot replace a pregnancy, which stimulates the growth of milk ducts and alveoli. Therefore, while you're producing milk, you may still be producing less milk than if you had been pregnant, which is why supplementing by feeding tube may be necessary. (For more on this, see chapter 6.)

Expect to provide at least some breast milk for the baby's nutritional needs, but it's rare to be able to produce enough milk to forego supplementing completely.

Remember that nursing an adopted baby not only depends on all the factors discussed in chapter 4, such as positioning and latch, but on the adopted baby's *willingness* to nurse.

In addition, unlike a birth mother's, your breasts may not respond well to stimulation, even if you've been taking a lactagogue and pumping for several months. An induced milk supply tends to build very slowly, reaching peak periods and drought periods.

Create Different Goals

When you're breastfeeding an adopted baby, it may not be possible to build a full or even partial breast milk supply, so you'll need to set different goals from a breastfeeding birth mother. In this case, you're breastfeeding to help establish a nursing relationship and to provide your baby with as much breast milk as possible, because some breast milk is certainly better than no breast milk.

Body Changes after Induced Lactation

As in any lactating woman, breast stimulation may interrupt your ovulation cycle and may change your breasts. So don't be surprised by the following:

- Changes in your menstrual cycle. This may translate into irregular cycles, no periods, or interrupted ovulation. This may reduce your chances of getting pregnant, but don't count on it. If you do get pregnant while you're breastfeeding, you can just carry on. See chapter 10 for details.

- Breast and nipple changes. Your areola may darken or you may experience tender breasts and breast fullness.

 Colostrum leaking from your breasts when the milk production begins.

⯎

As you can see, life today means that many nursing mothers will need to express/pump their milk at least once in a while. But it is also important to know when supplementing your baby may be necessary, and then what method of supplementation will be best. While a feeding tube at the breast is preferable if you and the baby are together, several different methods are recommended if you're separated and the baby is left with a caregiver. With that in mind, you are urged to read the next chapter thoroughly.

chapter 6

WHEN TO SUPPLEMENT

Most every nursing mother worries whether her baby is getting enough milk. Unfortunately, because of a lack of information available to the average breastfeeder, it's easy to be convinced that your baby needs extra supplementation—even when he doesn't. Or to be convinced that the baby needs no supplementation—when in fact he does!

This chapter is designed to clear up the confusion and define what "enough" really means. Whether your baby has dry diapers or is in a neonatal intensive care unit, read on for everything you need to know about supplementing your newborn.

IS THE CUSTOMER SATISFIED?

It's hard to believe that we are capable of producing milk that will keep the baby 100 percent satisfied, but we can. Human milk is recommended as the main course for the baby's first year and as a side dish for the second year and beyond.

The best bet is to breastfeed exclusively for six months before offering any solids to the baby. Then you can gradually introduce solids into your child's diet, breastfeeding less and less until the baby is weaned. Some women will continue nursing—although much less often—until their children are well past two years old. And that's just fine.

Is Colostrum Enough?

As discussed in earlier chapters, colostrum, the "premilk" your baby receives before your mature breast milk comes in, contains a high concentration of nutrients and immune factors to protect your baby from infection in the first few months of life. But many women worry that colostrum isn't enough to satisfy a hungry baby because it amounts to a relatively small quantity of just a few teaspoons or so per feeding.

Less Is More

There is a very specific purpose to the small amount of colostrum as compared with the abundant supply of mature milk. By not feeling full, your baby will suckle more frequently, which will cause your breasts to produce more milk early on. Frequent feeding will also ensure that more colostrum passes through your baby's digestive system, which will prevent newborn jaundice. The more colostrum that passes through your baby's system, the more efficient the newborn's body becomes at "clearing out" bilirubin, the yellow pigment that results as the baby breaks down old red blood cells to make way for new ones. Bilirubin is the source of newborn jaundice. (Jaundice is discussed more in chapter 8.) Research has confirmed that babies who are fed more frequently in the first few days of life have significantly lower levels of bilirubin. This is because colostrum doubles as a laxative, stimulating the baby's bowels to expel bilirubin in the stool before it has a chance to be reabsorbed by the body. These frequent colostrum feedings also offer another major benefit to you: They prevent engorgement, discussed more in chapter 7.

Normal Breastfeeding Patterns

When it comes to the early weeks of breastfeeding, there are as many definitions of "normal" as there are words in a dictionary. Your girlfriend's baby will have a different feeding pattern than your cousin's baby, your sister's baby, and your mother's friend's daughter's baby! In fact, breastfeeding patterns vary as widely as childhood growth and development patterns. One baby may breastfeed every hour, while another may feed every three or four hours.

Disregard anything that suggests a definite feeding schedule for your baby. As discussed in chapter 4, baby knows best. Feed the baby on demand, for as long as she wants. Period. The only one who can answer such questions as "How often should I feed my baby?" or "When will the baby sleep through the night?" is your *baby*! And even then, your baby may develop different patterns as she grows.

What I Can Tell You . . .

Yes, it's normal for your baby to want to feed long and often in the first few days. Don't discourage this pattern. Babies on these schedules may want to nurse as much as a couple of hours on the breast and then sleep for two hours; nurse for a couple more hours and then sleep for two more hours. And so on. This kind of early newborn pattern soon adjusts into shorter nursing periods and longer sleeping periods as your milk comes in and the baby becomes more satisfied with each feeding.

Other newborns may want to nurse for only ten minutes or so and then sleep for half an hour; nurse another few minutes and sleep again. And so it goes until your milk comes in, when the baby will begin to nurse longer and sleep longer. Sometimes babies are not interested in nursing at all, and may want to just sleep! In this case, you may need to wake up the baby to breastfeed. (See the section on sleepy babies on page 117 in chapter 4). Generally speaking, aim to nurse every two hours by day and every three hours by night (a minimum of ten to twelve times in a twenty-four-hour period).

Again, the baby's feeding pattern may change as she develops. It's common, for example, for a baby to suddenly want to nurse more often or longer than usual, a sudden burst that's referred to as a "growth spurt" or "frequency day." And of course, the more frequently the baby nurses, the more milk you'll make to meet those needs. Babies tend to go through growth spurts at around two weeks, six weeks, and three months.

A Word about Switching Sides

When you need to keep the baby alert during feeding or the baby has a weak suck, switching sides frequently during a nursing is encouraged. But if breastfeeding is going well, it's important to allow the baby to finish your first breast before you switch. This will ensure that the baby ingests the creamier hindmilk that comes at the end of the feeding. This richer milk is what keeps the baby satisfied longer between feedings.

The "foremilk," which is the first milk that comes out at the beginning of a feeding, is more like skim milk; it's low-fat and watery. There's also more of it than the hindmilk. But as the baby feeds, the skim milk turns to 1 percent milk, then 2 percent milk, then homogenized milk, then half-and-half, and finally pure cream, which is what makes the baby full and happy. In short, as the breast is emptied, the volume of milk delivered decreases as the fat content increases.

Your baby has finished the first breast when she falls asleep and slides off or lets go and starts looking for more. This is the perfect time to burp and switch over to side two.

A Climate of Change

There are some exceptions to the foremilk/hindmilk composition. In very hot climates, the body automatically adds more water to the breast milk, and the hindmilk in this case may resemble the foremilk of a woman in an average climate. This is nature's way of preventing the baby from becoming dehydrated.

In very cold climates, the opposite happens, and the milk is far fattier than milk in average climates. In this case, the foremilk may resemble the hindmilk of a woman in an average climate. This is nature's way of insulating the baby from the harsh climate. By the way, the same woman will make either fattier or more watery milk, depending on where she's living or traveling.

Signs of Good Eatin'

The first clue to whether your baby is getting enough breast milk is her behavior during and after feeding. You know that your baby is nursing well if you notice:

- Swallowing during nursing, in a suck-swallow pattern discussed in detail in chapter 4, page 100. When this occurs, you know that your letdown reflex is working and that the baby is having a good feed.

ᴘᴀ Your breasts are full before nursing, and soft after nursing. (If your breasts are engorged before nursing, they may not be completely soft after nursing but will certainly be *softer*. See chapter 7 for more details.)

ᴘᴀ The baby is nursing at least eight or more times each twenty-four hours (or as often as she wants).

ᴘᴀ The baby is nursing as long as she wants.

ᴘᴀ Once the milk comes in, the baby is content after most feedings.

Don't Worry—There's a Perfectly Logical Reason
See if any of your concerns turn up here.

Q. My baby seems to want to nurse all the time. I'm worried it's a sign that I don't have enough milk.
A. Lots of babies like frequent feedings. Many times it's the baby's way of saying, "Hey, I *like* this!" So take it as a compliment and carry on. As long as your milk letdown reflex is working and your baby is peeing, pooping, and growing, your baby is getting enough to eat.

Frequent feeding is most likely to be your baby's way of saying, "I want more. I'll just keep suckling until we've got the fridge stocked the way I like it!" In other words, the more your baby feeds, the more milk you'll make. This *assures* you that the baby is getting enough milk.

Finally, it's not unusual for breastfed babies to be hungry again after perhaps only an hour after being fed. This is because human milk gets digested more quickly than formula. If this happens regularly, it's nature's way of creating lots of suckling in the early days to increase your milk supply. If a baby continues to nurse this frequently and your milk supply doesn't increase, you may not have enough milk. In this case, you'll need to rule out a bad latch or other factors that may be decreasing your milk supply, such as medications, herbs, smoking, and so on. (Some of these substances are discussed in chapter 2.) You might also see your doctor or an LC, who may be able to nail down the problem.

Q. My baby doesn't seem to be burping enough. Is this a problem?
A. Don't be alarmed if your baby doesn't burp as much as you think is necessary. Breastfed babies tend to swallow far less air than bottle-fed babies

and therefore may not need to burp as much. Nevertheless, it's often a good idea to burp the baby for about five minutes after each side, or until you get a good burp.

Q. My baby used to nurse about twenty minutes on each breast. Now she's down to ten or fifteen minutes per breast. Is this a sign that there isn't enough milk for her?
A. No, it's a sign that your baby is becoming more efficient at suckling. You've got plenty of milk, and the honeymoon is over; now the baby wants to eat and run! Again, as long as your letdown is working and you notice the signs discussed in the previous section, your baby is getting enough.

Q. My baby is very fussy, whether he's hungry or not. What should I do?
A. Many babies have a "fussy time" but are not necessarily "fussy at the breast" or "fussy babies." Fussy *times* will usually occur at about the same hour each day and may not have anything to do with hunger at all; the reason usually has more to do with surroundings, sleeping habits, diaper discomfort, and so on. A process of elimination is the way to work through this, experimenting until your baby's fussiness resolves. Consulting a doctor may be helpful in this case.

When your baby fusses only when at the *breast*, reasons can include poor position or latch (see an LC), inadequate or overactive letdown (see chapter 4), teething, a reaction to something you've eaten that is being excreted in the milk, or an underlying infection such as an ear infection.

A less common reason for fussiness at the breast is a pattern of interrupting the baby's feedings before he's finished, and not allowing him to feed as long as he wants. In this case, stopping a baby before the first breast is completely empty will prevent him from getting the creamier, more satisfying hindmilk at the very end of the feeding. Here the fussiness at the breast becomes a Pavlovian response; your baby is learning to associate the breast with a feeling of dissatisfaction. The fussiness is the baby's way of saying, "Not *this* again. Look, it's not working for me! Leave me alone!" The only way to break the pattern is to allow unlimited feeding time and let the *baby* tell you when he's finished.

When you seem to have just a plain fussy baby—no matter *what* you do—there are ways to deal with the problem, discussed in chapter 8.

Q. My breasts don't seem to leak milk the way I'm told they're supposed to. Is this a problem?

A. No. As long as you're letting down milk when your baby is feeding and you're noticing a suck-swallow pattern, you have enough milk. Leaking has nothing to do with whether you're producing enough milk, it's just something that happens to many women when they're beginning to breastfeed. (Turning off letdown is discussed in chapter 4.)

Q. When I first began breastfeeding, my breasts were always hard before a feeding, but now they've really softened. Is this a sign that my milk production has gone down?

A. No; as long as your breasts are fuller before a feed and softer after, and your baby is peeing, pooping, and growing, your milk production is now just right for your baby's needs. As your milk adjusts to your individual baby's schedule and appetite, your breasts will become softer as the weeks go by. In addition, much of the "hardness" and fullness many women experience at first is due to engorgement, which is discussed in chapter 7.

Q. I just can't seem to feel the tingling I'm supposed to when my milk lets down. Does that mean the reflex isn't working?

A. No; many women don't feel anything when their milk lets down. If you're noticing the suck-swallow pattern discussed in chapter 4 and above, and if your baby is thriving, don't worry. A lot of women can't feel their letdown reflex but can feel some of the other signs of letdown discussed in chapter 4 (pages 98 to 101), including leaking. In some cases, women can feel their letdown for the first few days of breastfeeding and then stop feeling it as time passes.

The only time to worry about not feeling the letdown is if the baby doesn't begin that suck-suck-swallow pattern within the first five minutes of feeding. Of course, if letdown were not occurring, your baby would not be satisfied after feeding, would not be gaining weight, and would not be peeing and pooing properly, either. These things are discussed next. (See chapter 4, for more information on poor letdown if you're worried about it.)

Q. If my baby likes a bottle after breastfeeding, is this a sign that she's not full enough after breastfeeding?

A. Yes! Every time you give a bottle like this to your baby, you reduce your own breast-milk supply. The bottom line is that once bottles are introduced, less breastfeeding will take place unless you express your milk. Now, as long as this is planned (in the case of weaning, for example), that's fine. Just make sure you know how it works, or you could wind up engorged, with a nipple-confused baby and everyone frustrated.

Mind Those Pees and Poops

As one doctor aptly put it, a baby who poops, pees, and grows is doing just fine. That's why it's important to keep track of wet diapers and bowel movements.

In the First Week

While a newborn is feeding on colostrum in the first two to three days of life, expect several wet diapers per day. Once your milk comes in after the third or fourth day, the baby should generate at least four or five wet and heavy disposable diapers, or six or eight wet and heavy cloth diapers per day. The urine should be pale and odorless and contain no crystals.

As for bowel movements, your baby should be having one after almost every feeding (six to ten per day). Anything less than two to three bowel movements within a twenty-four-hour period should be cause for suspicion. In fact, breastfed babies will not begin to have fewer bowel movements until they are at least three months old. (See below for more details.)

If you're not sure what "wet and heavy" means in terms of wet diapers, pour a quarter cup of water on a dry diaper and compare it with your baby's diaper. If your baby's diapers seem considerably lighter, the baby isn't peeing enough.

As for poops: In the first day or two after birth, you'll notice that the baby's stools resemble black tar. This tarry consistency is the meconium (the waste produced by the fetus), which the baby has been storing during his stay in the womb. As the colostrum moves through the baby's system and works its laxative magic, these black tarry stools pass through, after which the stools begin to change color and consistency.

Greenish black, greenish brown, brownish yellow, or just plain yellow are all normal shades of your baby's stools during the first few days of breastfeeding. If the green/mustard color persists after a week or so, consult your doctor. The consistency of the breastfed baby's first stools will be loose, resembling pea soup, with a relatively mild, sweet odor. Once the mature milk comes in, normal breast-milk stools call to mind yellow water and seeds.

As the Baby Grows

Once the baby reaches six weeks, the diapers get bigger but the number of wet cloth or disposables remains the same. This time, add another four ounces of water to that quarter cup you were using in the first week as a diaper baseline. As the baby's bladder grows in size, it's able to hold more urine. The color should still be pale, however, without much of an odor.

Bowel-movement frequency tends to diminish as the baby gets older. For example, after about three months, it is normal for breastfed babies to go several days between bowel movements. During periods of rapid growth, however, they'll eat, pee, and poop far more. For the most part, frequency *really* varies from two or more movements per day to once a week. The more infrequent the bowel movements are, the larger the stools should be. A once a week poop, for example, can be expected to overflow the sleeper and run out of the neck and armholes (should be soft and runny on a breastfed baby); it's a major production! If stools are small and infrequent, the baby may not be getting enough milk, and you should consult your doctor.

As the baby regains her birth weight, bowel movements increase in number and size, particularly as the baby continues to gain weight.

If you find it difficult to keep track, *write it down,* noting when you're feeding and when you're changing a diaper.

Weight Watching

At first, the baby may lose up to 10 percent of his birth weight during the first few days of life. This is due to a limited amount of colostrum (see the discussion above) as well as a shedding of excess "womb fluids" such as placental blood and meconium. But not all babies lose weight, especially second and third babies, whose mothers may be more skilled at breastfeeding and producing breast milk. If the baby does not lose this weight, don't worry about it; it probably means that the baby is feeding more frequently.

By the second week of life, the baby will have regained that birth weight or more, after which you can expect a gain of about eight ounces per week, or about two pounds per month. But it's important to note that breastfed babies consume about 25 percent fewer calories than a formula-fed baby, even though the weight gains are similar. That's because breast milk is a much more efficient way of feeding babies.

To get an accurate weight reading, make sure you weigh the baby naked. Avoid "before and after" weighings around feedings. To date, all studies have shown that this kind of test weighing is not a reliable method for gauging how well the baby is eating, unless an electronic scale is used; most home scales are simply not sensitive enough to record such tiny fluctuations. And even when special electronic scales are used, the data from one feeding aren't suitable for a test weight; the before-and-after weights need to be averaged over a number of feedings to be accurate.

TO SUPPLEMENT OR NOT TO SUPPLEMENT?

I'm probably not the only one who was horrified by that 1995 story aired on *20/20* (an ABC newsmagazine show), which reported on breastfed babies who suffered brain damage as a result of malnourishment. In fact, that report inspired this entire chapter. The bottom line is that the women in that report did *not* have the information they needed to gauge whether their babies were getting enough milk. But if you're reading this book, you do!

For example, in that report one set of parents contacted a La Leche League leader instead of a doctor. Obviously, a doctor is the most appropriate person to contact if you suspect your baby isn't thriving. Moreover, several methods of supplementation are available, the best of which is by feeding tube at the breast and the worst of which is bottle feeding, which can confuse the baby and make matters worse. (See the section on nipple confusion in chapter 4).

When It's Not Necessary

One last time: If your baby is breastfeeding frequently (at least every two to three hours); if she's peeing, pooping, and growing; and if you're noticing all the signs of good eating discussed earlier, there is no need to supplement with *anything* else—neither plain water, sugar water, nor formula.

Why?

Your baby needs to breastfeed frequently so your breasts can begin to make milk. Supplements during the early days will fill up the baby and screw up your milk production. Worse, if the baby fills up on sugar water, he won't get the necessary calories and may lose more weight than is recommended. Sugar water also predisposes a baby to jaundice (see chapter 8). And if any of these supplements involve fake nipples, the baby will become confused. (See chapter 4.)

Another huge problem with unnecessary supplements is that you'll become engorged unless you express/pump your milk (see chapter 5).

Supplementing Myths

A variety of myths abound disguised as valid reasons to supplement. Here are three of the most common:

Myth: "Supplementing will help to detect a possible T-E fistula."
Fact: Fistula refers to an abnormal tunnel that links two internal organs. A T-E fistula stands for tracheo (windpipe)-esphogeal (food pipe) fistula: an abnormal linking of the windpipe and the esophagus. Women are sometimes told to postpone breastfeeding when this is suspected. Plain or glucose water is then given to the baby before she is given a chance to breastfeed. However, if a T-E fistula is suspected, the best medicine is breastfeeding and colostrum. Since colostrum is a physiological secretion, it is far less irritating to the baby's throat and lungs than plain or sugar water or formula. By the way, T-E fistula occurs in only about 1 in 4,000 newborns.

Myth: "You need to supplement to prevent jaundice."
Fact: Nonsense. Colostrum will do the trick better than anything else, because it acts as a laxative and clears out bilirubin at lightening speed. To date, all research has concluded that supplements do *not* reduce bilirubin levels—and in fact can have the opposite effect and increase them! Newborn jaundice is discussed in more detail in chapter 8.

Myth: "*Since you have a 'sleepy baby,' supplementing is necessary to prevent dehydration.*"

Fact: If you have what's called a sleepy baby, you'll need to *wake up the baby to breastfeed.* This is discussed thoroughly in chapter 4, page 117.

Truth and Consequences

Here's what happens when your baby is unnecessarily supplemented in the hospital:

1. You're given a subliminal message that your breast milk is insufficient.

2. Convinced that your baby needs extra water or formula, you dutifully feed this stuff to your baby, who breastfeeds less and less because he's filled up on supplement and may even become "nipple confused" (see chapter 4).

3. Your milk supply begins to dwindle because—guess what—your baby isn't breastfeeding. The more your baby suckles, the more milk you make. The less your baby suckles, the less milk you make.

4. In order to fix what was never "broke" in the first place, you'll need to rebuild your milk supply by expressing your milk regularly (see chapter 5) and may even need to reteach your baby how to breastfeed.

5. In some cases, the baby never goes back to the breast, and you'll need to feed your baby your own milk using an alternative feeder (see Tools of the Trade on page 166).

Retraining a Bottle-Fed Baby to Accept the Breast

A newborn given a fake nipple too soon may not latch on properly to the breast again. The easiest way to retrain is to finger-feed in the breastfeeding position, using the latch rules in chapter 4 (with tongue down) before putting your finger in the baby's mouth. You can then switch to a feeding tube at the breast (see figure 6-1), and then gradually return to normal breastfeeding.

Another retraining schedule is first cutting the baby off from any kind of nipple (real or fake), then feeding with an alternate feeder (see below) such as a periodontal syringe, soft plastic eyedropper, spoon, small clear glass, or flexible bowl. The next day, you can offer the baby your breast for comfort only, while you continue the feedings with an alternate feeder. This may get the baby to accept the breast once again, until you gradually begin to breastfeed again.

When Supplementing Is Necessary

If your baby isn't thriving, it's necessary to supplement nourishment with (in order of best to worst):

- your own expressed breast milk

- banked or donor breast milk

- formula for long-term supplementation or 5 percent glucose water for short-term supplementation

The definition of "not thriving" boils down to one, some, or all of these signs:

1. The baby is not gaining weight (see the Weight Watching section above).

2. The baby is not urinating at all or enough (see the "pees and poops" section above).

3. The baby is not having any or enough bowel movements.

4. The baby is continuously crying—no matter what you do—and will not accept the breast (see chapter 8 for more details).

5. The baby has persistent diaper rash (caused by too acidic a urine) and/or the urine has a strong odor and/or is yellow rather than clear.

6. The baby's urine has crystals in it.

7. The baby's stools do not correspond to the color or consistency they should be as discussed on pages 156 to 157 above.

Under these circumstances, take your baby to a doctor. In some cases, your baby's health is directly related to breastfeeding problems such as poor latch, poor milk supply, poor suckling, not frequent enough nursings, or too short a nursing period. In these cases, you'll need to supplement by a feeding tube at the breast (if possible) until you've corrected the underlying breastfeeding problem. If you can't empty your breasts effectively from nursing, you can keep up your milk supply by expressing/pumping your milk (see chapter 5).

Vitamin Supplements

In some circumstances, your doctor may recommend supplementing certain infants with vitamins E, D, and K. These vitamins can be given orally, with eyedroppers if necessary.

Vitamin D is recommended as a supplement for low-birth-weight babies and breastfed toddlers who are either darker skinned or not exposed to a great deal of sunlight. (We get vitamin D from sunlight, as well as certain foods.) Colostrum is very rich in vitamin E and an important guard against anemia. Under certain circumstances (when feeding isn't going well, for example), vitamin E may be recommended as a supplement since it's so important in the first few days of the baby's development.

Getting Breast Milk into Premature Newborns

Not all premature newborns will require substitute feeding; some may be able to breastfeed. This depends on the baby's age, weight, and overall health. It's common, however, for premies to be given their mother's breast milk by gavage or other means until they're able to breastfeed on their own.

Under these conditions, the best recommendation is to begin to express your milk ASAP. Your baby can be fed your colostrum and mature milk either exclusively (if possible) or in conjunction with other supplements (preferably donor milk if you don't have enough) until it's possible to breastfeed exclusively. If your baby is very young, your own breast milk can be made richer by adding human milk fortifier.

Keep in mind, however, that if your baby is very weak, your concern about him may affect your breast milk supply or letdown, although this is rare.

If you're having trouble, a lactogogue should do the trick. But even if you need to feed the baby an artificial supplement (see next section), certainly some of your own milk or colostrum is better than nothing.

Feeding Your Premie

Most of the alternative feeding tools discussed at the end of this chapter are not appropriate feeding methods for premies weighing less than 3.3 pounds (1,500 grams), which amounts to about a thirty-week gestation.

A baby this small may also be at risk for other health problems. Because of this, many premies this size are fed intravenously or even nasally, through a nasojejunal tube designed to provide constant nourishment. Here, a continuous stream of milk is pumped through a small tube that sits inside the baby's nose and goes directly into the small intestine.

Larger premies (weighing more than 3.3 pounds) may also be fed through a nasogastric tube, which is similar to the nasojejunal tube but sends the milk directly to the baby's stomach. The nasogastric tube is used when the baby can handle larger amounts of milk at each feeding.

Occasionally, larger and stronger premies can be fed via a feeding tube or nursing supplementer. Studies done on extremely low birth weight infants show that breastfeeding is physiologically less stressful than bottle feeding and that a higher body temperature during breastfeeding warms up the infant.

On the Menu

According to neonatal experts and the Committee on Nutrition at the American Academy of Pediatrics, the best liquid to feed all premies—whether naturally, intravenously, or through one of the nasal tubes discussed above—is your own fresh colostrum, followed by your own fresh milk. The colostrum is particularly crucial to help boost a premie's immune system and prevent illness. And interestingly, research shows that milk from mothers who delivered prematurely is richer in antibodies than from mothers who deliver at term. As the premie grows, the preterm milk changes in consistency and becomes mature breast milk.

As discussed in chapter 5, freezing can destroy some of the nutrients in both colostrum and mature breast milk, which is why fresh is best. If your own milk is not available, donor or banked milk (which will have been frozen to meet with HIV-screening standards) is the next-best thing, which can be enriched with human milk fortifier. Failing that, some of your own milk enriched with a fortifier or one of the special premie formulas on the market is the route to take.

If you're feeding your baby part breast milk and part formula, it's better to offer a balanced mixture of both (50 percent human milk and 50 percent formula) at every feeding, rather than pure formula for one feeding followed by pure breast milk at the next. By mixing the two liquids together, the baby will not only benefit from the enzymes in human milk that aid in digestion but will get an immune boost every time. If possible, giving breast milk first and topping off with formula is the best solution.

When Can a Premie Breastfeed?

When a premie cannot breastfeed, it's usually because of a weak suck, caused by an underdeveloped nervous system. As the baby matures and grows stronger, the suck will improve and allow for effective breastfeeding. Most current studies conclude that as soon as the baby is strong enough to suckle, she should be breastfed. In the recent past, many mothers were told to bottle-feed a premie first, prior to breastfeeding, but this practice serves no purpose and only winds up being more stressful for both baby and you. Generally, a premie is ready to breastfeed if the following criteria are met:

- The baby is in good general health and there are no underlying health problems that will interfere with breastfeeding.

- The baby is strong enough to coordinate sucking, swallowing, and breathing.

- The baby seems to be tolerating the milk that's been offered so far.

- The baby is able to maintain a viable body temperature outside the neonatal unit.

If the infant is very tiny, you can request a nurse, doctor, or LC to monitor the baby while you breastfeed.

Most premies will need you to put your hand behind their heads for support. The transitional hold is usually the best position (see chapter 4), while switching breasts may not be advisable if the baby's size is particularly small, since repositioning and relatching may prove too stressful for the baby. In this case, let the baby feed well on one breast; then, if the infant still seems interested, switch. And if the baby doesn't fully empty your breasts at a feeding, express/pump to finish the job. (See chapter 5.)

Is the Premie Getting Enough?

Since you can't gauge whether a premie is thriving by observing the usual diaper patterns or weight guidelines for newborns at term, "uterus rules" in this case reign supreme. In other words, a premie is considered to be growing well if the weight gain mimics what he would exhibit in the uterus. While theoretically uterus rules make sense, many doctors find them unrealistic, because the nourishment the baby receives in a neonatal unit does not in any way mimic placental nourishment. In fact, many premies simply do not gain weight at these womb rates, no matter what they eat.

When the baby is strong enough to go home, you can then use the same diaper and weight-gain guidelines as you would for a newborn at term. (See the Mind Those Pees and Poops and Weight Watching sections on pages 156 to 158.)

Multiples

Since it's more difficult with multiples to keep track of which baby is feeding when and which baby peed and pooped when, it's important to keep a journal and record each baby's feeding times, wet diapers, bowel movements, and weights. The rules regarding the number of wet diapers, frequency of bowel movements, and consistency of stools and urine do not change. You just have more babies to keep track of.

In many cases, some siblings thrive more than others. A number of factors can contribute to this, particularly if some siblings were kept in the hospital. Other contributing factors include restrictive hospital rules where only one baby is brought to you at a time, or when nighttime nursing is restricted. If you are separated from one baby who needs extra care, the other one will often thrive more. Finally, one baby may take to the breast better than another due to weak suck or a variety of problems discussed in chapter 4.

TOOLS OF THE TRADE

Okay, you need to supplement. But before you reach for that baby formula, remember *this* one: supplementation = formula + bottle.

Since most cases involving supplementing are temporary, it's important to choose your supplementing tools wisely. Opt for a tool that will not interfere with natural breastfeeding and will allow your baby to continue to suckle on your breast.

A variety of supplementing tools are available: cup, bowl, spoon, eyedropper, periodontal syringe, feeding tube at the breast, or nursing supplementer. A bottle, of course, is also available, but will interfere with natural breastfeeding if the baby is too young or hasn't yet had six weeks of good breastfeeding. Whatever method you choose, make sure you discuss it with your baby's doctor.

Feeding Tube

When you cross a bottle with a nursing supplementer (discussed next), you get a special pediatric feeding tube that can be placed into a regular baby bottle.

Here you put your supplement in a regular baby bottle, put the feeding tube through the regular hole in the nipple, and cut an extra hole in the bottle nipple to let air in (see figure 6-1).

Finger-Feeding with the Tube

Hold the baby in a breastfeeding position and slip the feeding tube into the baby's mouth with your finger alongside the rubber nipple, until the end of the tube is about at the end of the nipple. Your finger should be positioned with the nail side up in the baby's mouth, about two joints in. Nurse on that side until half the bottle is empty; then switch to the other side until the baby seems to be full.

Figure 6-1
BREASTFEEDING WITH THE TUBE

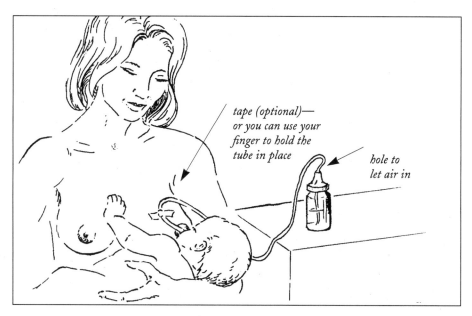

tape (optional)—or you can use your finger to hold the tube in place

hole to let air in

Illustration by Karen Leiser, 1995.

Breastfeeding with the Tube

If you're using this method to train the baby to latch onto the breast correctly (as shown in figure 6-1), you would either tape the tube onto your breast and latch the baby, or else latch the baby onto the breast first and then slip in the tube. Eventually, you would simply remove the tube without the baby noticing and let the baby feed on your nipple when your letdown has occurred. Or if you're using this method to supplement a regular feeding, just breastfeed as usual and introduce this feeding tube after your breasts are emptied and let the baby feed until she's full.

The Advantages

This method helps train your baby to take the breast and is also more portable than the nursing supplementer. The tube will cost under two dollars and will not lead to nipple confusion. This is definitely the method of choice in any short-term situation. A longer-term situation may require a nursing supplementer, which is more difficult to master.

Figure 6-2
A Nursing Supplementer

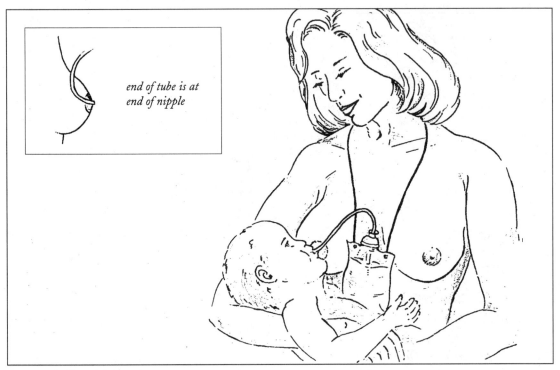

*end of tube is at
end of nipple*

Illustration by Karen Leiser, 1995.

Nursing Supplementer

A nursing supplementer, the next-best thing to natural breastfeeding, is often used to train a baby to breastfeed if that baby was confused by a fake nipple too early in the game.

This product has a plastic bag or bottle that contains the supplement, which hangs on a cord around your neck, resting between your breasts. A long, thin tube is attached to the container with its open end taped to your breast, extending about a quarter of an inch past your nipple (see figure 6-2).

Models come with different sizes of tubing; the larger the tubing, the faster the milk flows. The choice depends largely on the baby's ability to suck and why you're supplementing to begin with, but it's a good idea to start with medium tubing. You can also ask your doctor about which tubing size is appropriate.

Where you place the supplement container will also help determine how fast the milk flows. The higher the supplement container is placed on your body, the faster the flow. When the bottom of the supplement container is above your nipple, the milk will flow out nonstop, which can cause the baby to choke. The lower the container is placed, the harder the baby will need to suck in order to get the milk.

As in normal breastfeeding, good positioning and latch-on are important. If the baby opens his mouth wide when going onto the breast and takes the breast far back into the mouth, he'll learn to breastfeed correctly while stimulating your milk supply. But if the baby sucks on the tip of your nipple along with the tubing, you may wind up with sore nipples owing to a poor latch. (Sore nipples are discussed in chapter 7.)

Finally, make sure that when you tape the tubing to your breast the tape is near the edge of your areola and not too close to the nipple. Once you're all taped up, then hold the baby in any of the breastfeeding positions discussed in chapter 4 and let the baby suck from the tube in much the same way as you would from a straw.

Some supplementer models have a tie-off cap that keeps the milk from flowing until the baby actually sucks (but you must loosen it to feed). Others are "double breasted," including two tubes that you can tape to both breasts to make it easier to switch sides or even feed multiples. With the two-tube system, you pinch one tube until the baby latches, then let go; the second tube is the air intake. Here are further instructions:

1. Place the tube near the center of the baby's upper lip. You can also use your own nipple to touch the baby's lip. The goal is to get the baby to open her mouth.

2. When the baby grasps the breast and tube together, wait for jaw compression, then push down slightly on the supplementer bottle to reward the baby's sucking with a small dribble of fluid.

3. If the baby stops sucking, keep her interested by allowing more fluid to fall on her lips.

The Advantages

Nursing supplementers essentially teach both you and the baby how to breastfeed by letting the baby stimulate milk production while receiving the supplement. A baby sucking on the tube is also sucking on your nipple, helping to establish your milk supply. You can also walk around while you're feeding, which you can't do with any other method.

If the baby cannot take the breast (for any number of reasons), you can still use the nursing supplementer for feeding by taping the tubing to your index finger and introducing it gently (pad side pushing on tongue) into the baby's mouth. When finger-feeding, the baby also uses his mouth and tongue properly.

The Disadvantages

The nursing supplementer is the most expensive and complicated kind of feeding equipment, costing roughly forty U.S. dollars. It's also not as portable or convenient as the other methods available, and some women report that the skin on their areola gets irritated from the tape. In this case, either purchase hypoallergenic tape or just put the tube in and forget about taping.

In some cases, the babies get so used to the continuous, steady flow of milk provided by the tubing, they may refuse to breastfeed when the tubing is removed. The solution here is to intermittently pinch the tube once letdown has occurred to ease the baby onto full, natural breastfeeding.

And as in all cases in which you're using another system to feed the baby, some mothers become dependent on the reassurance that the artificial system provides; they can actually see the milk flowing into the baby's mouth. This makes some women hesitant to breastfeed naturally. Review the Is the Customer Satisfied? section on page 149 to gauge whether the baby is getting enough milk once breastfeeding resumes naturally.

Things to Keep in Mind

If after using the nursing supplementer for a few weeks, there is no improvement in a baby's weak suck, ask to see an LC, who may recommend an occupational therapist or physical therapist trained in neurodevelopment and breastfeeding to evaluate the baby more carefully.

The nursing supplementer is designed with a built-in discontinuation factor. In other words, as the baby's suck improves and your milk supply goes up, the baby gets less milk from the supplementer. Discontinuing the use of the tube then is automatic.

If you seem to have difficulty getting the baby to nurse without the supplementer, try a smaller tubing size, or put less supplement into the container.

In a few cases, babies cannot be persuaded to nurse without the supplementer and will insist on it until they can drink from a cup.

Cup-Feeding

Cup-feeding is growing in popularity in North America. In Kenya and Tanzania, a baby born prematurely and not yet ready for breastfeeding, or a baby separated from his mother, will always be cup-fed rather than bottle-fed. In fact, throughout East Africa, nipple confusion is unheard of, since bottles are never used.

To cup-feed properly, you'll need a small cup or shot glass, or even a flexible bowl. There's no special cup you need to purchase; any clean cup, glass, or bowl will do. By going slowly with the following directions, any baby should be able to use a cup or bowl:

1. Hold the baby upright.

2. Place a small amount of your supplement in the cup, glass, or bowl.

3. Gently tilt the cup or bowl to the baby's lips, letting just a small amount of liquid into the baby's mouth.

4. As with spoon-feeding, allow the baby to completely swallow before offering more.

The Advantages
Cup-feeding is cheap, effective, portable, and convenient. Nor does it interfere with breastfeeding, since the baby acquires the same tongue-thrust habit.

Spoon-feeding

Spoon-feeding was once considered to be a cheap feeding tool, one that did not interfere with breastfeeding. But experts really discourage spoon-feeding on the grounds that it is simply an extremely inefficient way to feed a baby. It takes too long, and you need a very patient baby to actually nourish him or her adequately with this feeding method.

Eyedropper or Periodontal Syringe

In the same way that you would use an eyedropper to feed a baby animal, you can feed a tiny baby. Eyedroppers or periodontal syringes (aka orthodontic syringes) are usually employed when feeding a premature baby. The best kinds are made of soft, unbreakable plastic. The only difference between an eyedropper or a syringe is that the syringe holds more fluid; the feeding technique, however, is identical. Here are the instructions:

1. Sit the baby straight up in your lap, chin tucked down toward chest to prevent choking or aspirating fluid.

2. Put the eyedropper or syringe to the baby's mouth and gently drip the milk in.

3. Make sure the baby swallows completely before you offer more.

The Advantages
This may be particularly effective for tiny premature babies who cannot yet breastfeed, though equipment must be purchased which varies in cost. But it is a method both convenient and portable, and it does not interfere with breastfeeding because it does not teach the baby a different sucking style.

Bottle

Last—and probably least in this case—is a bottle. Bottles are bad ideas if the baby hasn't yet had at least six weeks of good breastfeeding. If the baby is under three months old and you need to temporarily supplement but fully intend to go back to breastfeeding, avoid bottle-feeding at all costs.

Aside from this, bottle-feeding is a perfectly easy and portable way to feed your baby. Long nipples (such as Nuks) tend to be better because they can help to reduce nipple confusion in case you want to breastfeed again, though they cannot guarantee it.

✍

In many cases, supplementing is necessary not so much because of the baby's health but your own. If, for example, nursing is persistently painful, supplementing the baby with one of the methods discussed above may be necessary until you track down the origin of your pain—be it sore nipples or deep breast pain. The next chapter discusses all the reasons why nursing may hurt, and what you can do to heal yourself and your breastfeeding experience.

chapter 7

WHEN NURSING HURTS

A s I've been saying, anytime you're in physical pain or discomfort during breastfeeding, it's a sign that something's *wrong*. When nursing hurts, there is *always* a reason; and in order for you to continue breastfeeding comfortably, the source of the hurt must be investigated and, if possible, treated. Occasionally, women who don't want to continue breastfeeding will use "it hurts too much" as an excuse to stop. And this is an excuse that many doctors have and still do support. But think about what you might do if, for example, urinating suddenly began to "hurt" too much. Would you just stop urinating without investigating the source of the pain, and, if possible, treating the pain? Of course not! So why would you stop breastfeeding? You can continue to express your milk to keep up your milk supply until the source of your pain is treated, and then feed your baby another way until you feel comfortable with suckling again. But to simply stop the process altogether and allow your milk to dry up is a most unfortunate decision, particularly if the source of your pain is easily detected and rectified.

This chapter discusses every possible source of pain during breastfeeding, from the most common—engorgement, mastitis, and plugged ducts—to the more obscure. I also examine other breast problems, including breast lumps and cysts.

I'M STUFFED: ENGORGEMENT

Feeding early and frequently at birth helps prevent engorgement, or being overfilled or stuffed with milk. Although most doctors will tell you that engorgement is normal, lactation consultants maintain that it's caused by poor breastfeeding management, poor latch, and/or not feeding often or long enough. In other words, with proper instruction after birth, engorgement is preventable.

When your baby takes to the breast right after birth, and begins nursing frequently on colostrum, you will most likely not become engorged. But if you encounter any of the numerous problems discussed in chapters 4, 5, and 6, such as poor latch, separation from the child for some reason, and so on, you may indeed become engorged unless you're regularly emptying your breasts. Engorgement is painful and may cause the tissue around the nipple to be swollen, and hence flat. The pain of engorgement is caused by an increased blood supply to the breast, combined with an accumulation of milk. This spells trouble for the breastfeeding novice and can frustrate the baby, who may have an incredible instinct to suckle. The less often you nurse, the worse engorgement is; the better you are at making milk, the worse it is too. The good news is that should you fall prey to engorgement, it's only temporary. Emptying your breasts of the milk and continuing to frequently empty your breasts is the general cure.

When to Expect Engorgement

Unfortunately, engorgement is a common experience on the second or third day after birth. This is why, if your hospital stay extends beyond a day or so, it's so important to request rooming-in privileges and to make sure that your hospital is "baby friendly" (see chapter 3). Engorgement will be less severe if your baby has access to your breast at all times, but hospitals with centralized nurseries and scheduled feedings do not encourage this, and severe engorgement is subsequently common. This is often the case if the hospital has an ongoing arrangement with baby formula companies ("We'll give you money if you push our formula.") That's why it's important to read chapter 3 and put breastfeeding on your birth plan! It's also worth noting that our mothers and grandmothers who may have told us that they "tried breastfeeding but it was too painful" were probably engorged and never given an opportunity to *relieve* the engorgement. Instead, they were told that some women just "can't" breastfeed and were instructed by their doctors to switch to formula.

In hospitals where breastfeeding is taken seriously, engorgement is considered sufficient cause to file an incident report, because it indicates that you have not received proper care. This report then mars a hospital employee's record for the duration of that person's career.

Engorgement is also a common problem if you're separated from your baby due to illness (yours or the baby's), for example, and do not start regular pumping right away. This is particularly true in cases where you've prematurely delivered, or *any* other time you are not able to empty your breasts as frequently or efficiently as you should.

Here are the most common scenarios in which infrequent or insufficient breast emptying occurs:

- *When the baby has a poor latch.* A baby who isn't latched onto the breast properly will not be able to empty the breast sufficiently. This is particularly common during the first week of breastfeeding. If this problem isn't corrected, your milk supply will begin to dwindle. See chapter 4 for more details.

- *When you've got a bad pump.* Sometimes the road to hell is paved with pumps from hell. If you're pumping, make sure you invest in a good pump. Review chapters 3 and 5 for more details.

- *When you've been using a "booby trap" such as nipple shields.* Chapter 3 discusses these terrible inventions in detail.

- *When you're going back to work.* You know you need to empty your breasts, but your work environment isn't mother friendly. Check out chapter 9 for some suggestions on how to breastfeed in the workplace.

- *When you're deliberately weaning.* When you wean too quickly, your milk supply may not get the message to taper off, and so you may become engorged. In this case, the answer is simple: Empty your breasts regularly just a little bit until you're comfortable. Chapters 9 and 10 discuss weaning in more detail.

What to Expect When You're Engorged

Essentially, being engorged feels exactly as it sounds: congested and over-filled. Milk may leak out of your breasts and, if you're not wearing a proper nursing bra, spill down your shirt. Your breasts and armpit area will feel swollen, hard, and sore. When you're engorged, letdown can feel something akin to your arms being ripped out of their sockets; in other words, it HURTS!

Engorgement ranges from mild to severe. When you're suffering from severe engorgement, the tissue around the nipple and areola becomes so hard and tight the baby can't even grasp the nipple, and so pulls away and cries in frustration. Or the baby gets only the end of the nipple, which may damage the nipple and won't allow the breast to be emptied effectively. Engorgement may lead to a plugged duct, mastitis, or even a breast abscess. These are discussed farther on.

How Do You Spell R-E-L-I-E-F?

Emptying the breasts of milk is the first step in treatment. If poor latch is causing the engorgement, you'll need to get the milk out by self-expressing or pumping (see chapter 5) and work with a doctor or lactation consultant to correct the latch problem before you put the baby back on the breast (see chapter 4).

If latch is not a problem, the baby is the best breast emptier around, but sometimes you may need to express/pump some milk yourself to soften up the area around the nipple before putting the baby onto your breast. If you're severely engorged, your doctor can recommend an appropriate painkiller to help you. Another option is to request an oxytocin nasal spray (discussed in chapter 4), which will help with milk letdown (your letdown may not work as well when you're in pain), which will speed up breast emptying.

No Limits
The *worst* thing you can do when your breasts are engorged is to limit nursing times (an impulse when you're in pain), which only makes engorgement worse. Unlimited breastfeeding, on the other hand, relieves engorgement

and prevents future engorgement episodes. After the initial pain of letdown, nursing feels better. Nursing for only short periods of time will actually make matters worse, resulting in pain without gain! Resist the urge to skip your nursings or procrastinate nursing because it's painful. You know what happens when you do this? More engorgement. The only way to relieve your breasts is to nurse, nurse, nurse.

Soothing Suggestions

- If expressing your milk prior to feeding is difficult, a warm shower will help with milk letdown.

- Soothe yourself with whatever works. Whether it's ice packs, warm towels (mothers have been known to heat wet washcloths in the microwave and then apply them), hot baths, or showers, do it. Chilling big cabbage leaves and wearing them inside your bra is reportedly helpful—but only if you remove them within four hours; otherwise, you may notice lowered milk production as some women have reported.

Preventing Engorgement

To avoid repeating the engorgement experience, keep on breastfeeding as much and as often as the baby likes. Avoid giving the baby an artificial nipple until she's been breastfeeding well for at least six weeks. (See the section in chapter 4 on nipple confusion.) And anytime you've skipped a nursing for any reason, replace it with an expressing/pumping session (see chapter 5 for more details).

IT'S MASTITIS UNTIL PROVEN OTHERWISE

Breasts and nipples are like any other part of the body: They can get infected too! Antibiotics will fix this. The most common breast infection is called *lactational mastitis,* meaning infection of the milk-producing breast. This happens during breastfeeding and affects as many as 10 percent of the breastfeeding population. Bacteria (usually staphylococcus, sometimes streptococcus—normal skin bacteria we all carry around with us) gets inside the breast through the nipple.

Lactational mastitis is sometimes preceded by a plugged milk duct (discussed farther on), but plugged ducts don't necessarily mean you've got mastitis. In other words, although plugged ducts can occur when you don't have mastitis, they are sometimes a symptom of it.

Before the days of antibiotics and short postdelivery hospital stays, mastitis epidemics often struck hospitals and occurred far less often away from the hospital. The epidemic form of mastitis is rarely seen anymore, due to a radical change in postpartum health practices.

It Feels Like the Flu

One family doctor told me that any nursing mother who thinks she has the flu has mastitis until proven otherwise. That's because the initial symptoms of mastitis are fatigue and a flulike, muscular aching. This is usually followed by a fever, a rapid pulse, and the development of a hot, reddened, tender area on the breast. Sore nipples are not a symptom of mastitis, although it's possible to have sore nipples and mastitis. (Sore nipples are discussed in the next section.) When a fever and chills develop, the mastitis is probably more severe, and it's taking your entire body to fight off the infection.

If mastitis isn't treated properly, an abscess may develop. When a "walled off" portion of the breast gets bluish red, swollen, and inflamed, this is a classic sign that an abscess is in the making; it might need to be drained via a needle, or a tiny incision in the breast. "Walling off" means that your immune system has walled off the infectious area, allowing the rest of your body to carry on as usual.

While mastitis usually occurs in only one breast, it's not unusual to see a double-breasted infection. In some cases, mastitis can also affect the composition of the milk, increasing levels of sodium and chloride. This is probably your body's way of protecting the baby from infection.

Mastitis most often occurs about five weeks into breastfeeding and lasts between two and four days so long as it's treated. It's crucial that you not stop breastfeeding when you have mastitis; this could lead to an abscess.

Types of Mastitis

There are several kinds of mastitis, and they're classified according to where in the breast they're located and by the symptoms you suffer. Remember that the suffix *itis* (pronounced eye-tiss) simply means "inflammation."

Cellulitis

This refers to inflammation of the cellular breast tissue. (No—it's not "inflammation of cellulite"!) This means that the lobular, connective tissue inside your breast (see chapter 1) is infected. In cellulitis, infection starts in the breast tissue; bacteria enters the breast through a break in the skin (usually through a cracked nipple), and the condition is seen in the first weeks of breastfeeding rather than later on. The symptoms of cellulitis include general ill health (fatigue, aches) and a headache, while a warm, tender reddened area of the breast may also develop. Pus rarely forms with cellulitis.

Adenitis

This is an inflammation of the ducts within the breast. Here the infection starts in the milk spaces due to poor emptying of part of the breast, resulting in milk "stasis," where the milk hangs around longer than it should. In this case, pus is more likely to form.

Subclinical Mastitis

This means mild mastitis. Here there are usually no symptoms other than a low fever. You may just feel like you have a touch of the flu or a cold.

Nonlactational Mastitis

In this bacterial breast infection in nonlactating women, bacteria gets deeper inside the breast somehow—via lumpectomy, immune deficiency, and so on. Diabetic women are prone to this for the same reasons they are prone to yeast infections. Here the breast can develop skin boils, accompanied by flulike symptoms. Antibiotics take care of this, too.

About Abscesses

The best way to prevent abscesses is to continue to breastfeed frequently, sore side first. The rules for preventing abscesses (and managing mastitis) are *heat, rest, empty breast*. Heat means warm compresses or a warm shower; rest means going to bed and staying there until you feel better (you take baby with you, by the way); emptying the breast means breastfeeding frequently. After nursing, express milk from the sore area (known as "stripping") to see if there's any pus in it; if there is, express milk after each nursing until the milk runs clear. If this is done, an abscess should not develop, and you may not even require antibiotics. Also, change positions frequently during feeding. This will help to empty all the milk sinuses and ductules in the breast.

If an abscess does occur, after "walling off" it will look like a localized white area just under the surface of the skin, which will feel very warm and tender when you touch it. Treatment with antibiotics and possibly draining the abscess (after making an incision) may be necessary. (Treatment of mastitis is discussed further on.)

The problem with an abscess is that you may need to temporarily stop breastfeeding, because the infection can be passed on to the baby. In this case, you would pump your milk but *discard* it instead of feeding it to the baby. You'll need to supplement with formula or donated breast milk until you can resume breastfeeding. On rare occasions, an abscess may cause a puslike discharge from your nipple. In any event, once the infections clears (and it will), you should be able to carry on as usual.

Who Gets Mastitis?

Some women are more prone to mastitis than others. Studies show that the following can predispose you to it:

- *A decrease in nursing.* When you're nursing less frequently than usual, this causes more milk to sit around in the ducts.

- *Engorgement.* When you're engorged, you're more likely to develop a bacterial infection because, again, milk sits around longer in your ducts.

- *Stress.* Half the women who suffered from mastitis and were surveyed by La Leche League in a 1980 study stated that they'd been under some sort of stress prior to its onset. Stress comes from anything from overwork to fatigue—above and beyond what's considered normal when looking after an infant. As a result, the term *holiday mastitis* has been coined, because the cure—lots of rest, among other things—forces you to take a holiday.

- *Cracked nipples.* This creates a wonderful transmission route for the bacteria! The key to avoiding sore nipples is to ensure that your baby is latched on correctly (see chapter 4).

- *Tight bras or tops.* These reduce breast emptying because they compress milk ducts. Milk that isn't emptied can become infected.

- *Sleeping facedown.* Again, this compresses milk ducts, resulting in poor breast emptying.

- *Using nipple shields.* If you're using a nipple shield because of sore nipples (discussed next), you will not be able to effectively suckle and empty your breast, thus causing mastitis.

- *Poor diet*—particularly one low in iron, which causes anemia.

Treating Mastitis

Depending on how severe your symptoms are, antibiotics may be necessary. For cellulitis, any antibiotic that can handle staphylococcus, which is also safe to use during breastfeeding, is fine. For adenitis, the drug of choice is erythromycin because it penetrates into the milk spaces where the infection is. While penicillin and ampicillin used to be old standbys, many strains of staphylococcus are now resistant to them. When antibiotics are used and breastfeeding is continued, the mastitis will be cured within forty-eight hours.

If your mastitis symptoms seem to be less severe, antibiotics may not be necessary. Following the rules outlined above for preventing abscesses (and hence severe mastitis) is the best medicine for managing mastitis: *heat, rest, empty breast.* If you have adenitis, stripping the pus from the affected breast is necessary too. Often mastitis will simply clear up on its own.

Self-Help

Of course, you may feel quite ill with mastitis, especially if you're running a high fever. In this case, here are the rules:

1. Rest in bed. Take the baby in with you as long as you don't have a waterbed or share the bed with someone who is drunk, stoned, or who weighs over 300 pounds.

2. Nurse as frequently as you can for as long as the baby obliges. This will help to clear out the milk from the ducts, which will help your body fight off the infection.

3. If you're sore, apply moist heat to the affected area of the breast (if you have a reddened area). Warm, wet towels or washcloths are better than heating pads.

4. If you have a fever, drink lots of fluids to prevent dehydration.

5. If you're on antibiotics, take them as prescribed by your physician, or else their effect will be compromised. Even though you may start to feel better before the infection is completely gone, *finish the course of treatment*. Stop too early, and you increase the chances of recurrence.

PULLING THE PLUG: PLUGGED DUCTS

If you develop a sore lump in one area of the breast but don't seem to have a fever, you probably have a plugged duct, also known as the "plug." This usually refers to ducts plugged at the nipple level, but a plug can also occur higher up in the breast, often the result of scarring or constriction instead of thickened milk, which causes the plug around the nipple. A plug higher up is referred to as an obstructed duct.

In either case, the soreness occurs because a duct isn't draining properly and has therefore become inflamed. Pressure builds up behind the plug, causing inflammation in the surrounding tissues. This is also sometimes referred to as "caking," and it usually occurs in only one breast. A milk duct will plug up when milk sits around the ducts too long as a result of engorgement, breast constriction, or insufficient breast-emptying. The result may be that less milk flows out of the nipple.

Many of the same triggers of mastitis are at work here, but some women just seem to be prone to chronic plugs, for reasons not yet known. And, of course, plugged ducts will often *cause* mastitis. What we do know is that women tend to be plagued by plugs during the winter, due to heavier and more restrictive clothing.

What Should You Do?

Breastfeed like mad. The suckling may help to dislodge the plug and allow the milk to flow normally. Also use your "mastitis rules" and apply moist heat to the area several times a day as soon as you notice symptoms (review the section on mastitis above).

In addition, massage the breast to help stimulate the flow of milk, very effective in a hot shower or bath. When massaging, use the palm of your hand and all your fingers in a gentle but firm circular motion, starting behind the lump and working toward the nipple. To help loosen the plug, breastfeed the baby or express some milk right after treating the sore area with warmth and massage. "Stripping" the breast may also help (see further above), and once again, change positions frequently during feeding.

When to Contact a Doctor
See your doctor immediately if any of the following apply:

- You're feeling sick (especially if you're running a fever or vomiting).

- You're not feeling sick, but rest, heat, nursing and stripping breasts (if there's pus) haven't made things better within twenty-four hours.

- Your nipple is dry and patchy.

- Blood or pus is in your milk or is discharging from the nipple.

- There are any red streaks near the sore area.

These are all signs of either a bacterial infection or a more severe infection at work.

WHEN IT'S JUST PLAIN SORE NIPPLES

Whether you have normal, flat, or inverted nipples, the most common cause of sore nipples is a poor latch (see chapter 4). Poor latch subjects the nipple to traction and friction, resulting in soreness, stripes, bruises, abrasions, cracks, and even craters. "Cliff-hanging," when most of the areola is not in the baby's mouth and the baby is suckling on the nipple only, is a classic problem that can be easily fixed. When you have a red vertical stripe on the nipple, this is a sign that the baby is chewing or gumming the nipple. It may also indicate a poor tongue-thrust habit.

Sore nipples have a domino effect on breastfeeding: The sorer you are, the less you breastfeed, the less milk you make, and the more frustrated everyone becomes. So the first step in investigating the cause of your sore nipples is to make sure that the baby is latched on correctly. You must also do the following:

- Use a modfied lanolin cream, such as Lansinoh, which can help heal cracked, sore nipples, and prevent dryness and scab formation.
- Rinse your bras out with vinegar to eliminate any laundry soap residue, and then rinse them out a second time with clear water.
- Make sure that when you apply cologne, deodorant, hair spray, shampoo, conditioner, or powder you don't involve the nipple area.

If a poor latch is the problem, your soreness will develop in the first week or two of breastfeeding. In this case, you must fix the latch. You will know when you have a good latch, because whatever discomfort you feel will improve after the first few minutes of nursing. If you're too sore, consult a lactation expert about proper latch-on. With a good latch, the problem should immediately resolve. If you can't see someone right away, you may need to express or pump your milk for a few days (see chapters 5 and 6) and then put the baby on the breast in a correct latch before continuing with breastfeeding.

If the soreness does not improve after three days of consistently working to correct the latch, your baby may have a sucking problem. In this case, consult your baby's doctor to identify the problem and learn how to correct it or feed the baby despite it. This is discussed in detail in chapter 4, in the Mouths of Babes section.

But I *Checked* the Latch!

If the baby is latched on correctly but your sore nipples persist, then clearly your soreness is caused by something else. In this case, it's important to keep track of how long the pain or soreness lasts after feeding begins.

Soreness that lasts throughout the feeding can indicate a variety of problems, such as a fungal infection (see farther on); bad breast pads (see chapter 3); or an allergy—to wool, for example, if you're wearing sweaters without a bra or using a lanolin-based cream, or to a soap or nipple cream you're using. If your baby has started solids, residue from some foods may also irritate the skin on your nipples.

If you suspect an allergy is the culprit, try to self-isolate the irritant through the process of elimination. Itchiness usually means wool. Remember, too, that nipples need air, light, and dry fabrics near them. If you're leaking, consult chapter 4, page 122, to learn how to turn off letdown, and change your clothing or breast pads more frequently until you've mastered this technique. Apparently, wire tea-strainers worn inside your bra will hold your clothing away from your nipples and allow for more air circulation.

A Word about Sunshine

Almost every book on breastfeeding will tell you that direct sunlight is the best source of light for your nipples. Maybe this worked in 1976, but not today! The risk of UV damage is too great. Don't do this, and disregard any book section that gives directions on how much sun to take in or suggests you use a "UV lamp."

Don't Go Anywhere Near . . .

- Nipple shields (see the Booby Traps section in chapter 3).
- Breast shells (see chapter 3).

ɤ Ointments containing antibiotics, steroids, astringents, or anesthetic agents (these may even numb the nipples, interfering with letdown).

ɤ Hair dryers to infected nipples. (This is okay if there is no infection.)

When It's a Skin Thing

Nipples are covered with skin, which, like skin anywhere else on your body, can get dry, cracked, and itchy from rashes, or even eczema (if you have eczema on other parts of your body, for example).

Rashes

The most common rash is caused by frequent skin contact between your baby's mouth and your nipple. Something is irritating your nipples, perhaps even residue of solid foods your baby is eating. This is a rash that rarely needs medical treatment and clears up by keeping the nipple clean, dry, and exposing it to indoor light. If a mild rash or dry skin persists, see your doctor. There is a rare kind of breast cancer, known as Paget's disease that is characterized by a rash or dryness around usually one nipple.

If the rash on the nipple causes scaling on other areas of the breast, and if you notice scaling on other body parts such as the scalp, elbows, or knees, you'll definitely need to see a doctor to rule out psoriasis. If you do have it, treatment usually involves a topical cream containing 1 percent hydrocortisone, which you'll need to use between feedings and wipe off prior to breastfeeding.

If you have nipple damage of some kind, Raynaud's syndrome can develop, where the nipple turns white and is extremely sensitive during and after feedings. The cure for this is finding the source of the damage (usually a bad latch) and fixing it. A painkiller safe to use during breastfeeding will help until the nipples heal.

Breast Herpes

If you've been exposed to the herpes simplex virus (HSV), you can develop herpes sores on your nipples. Most doctors will be able to determine if you have a herpes simplex sore (called a vesicle) just by visual inspection, but a culture will confirm it.

HSV I or II can now be associated with sores above the waist. (In the past, HSV II was the dreaded genital herpes, but now it's seen above the waist, too.) Anytime you have a cold sore or fever blister, it's a sign that HSV is active. In this case, the nipple and areola can also be sites for these sores. If this is your diagnosis, you may need to wean your baby until the virus has cleared up, pumping your breasts and feeding the baby your milk with another feeding tool (see chapters 5 and 6).

The symptoms of breast herpes are characterized by extreme pain during breastfeeding. The sores must be kept dry, however, and in this case, dusting them with cornstarch and blow-drying them may be helpful. So long as the baby has been breastfeeding exclusively until now, the antibodies in your milk should provide protection from the virus. There is no cure for herpes, but the sores will go away and will reappear less and less frequenlty, until you will simply not be bothered by them anymore.

The Bleb

In rare cases, you'll notice a whitish, tender area ("bleb") under your areola, which looks like milk under the skin. This milk has somehow become trapped there, and it will cause the nipple and areola to become inflamed. An extremely painful condition, it can take several days or weeks to heal. The cure for the bleb is time; you need to wait for new skin to replace the old skin. Eventually, the bleb is exposed as the old skin cells slough off.

Until the bleb goes away, your doctor may need to aspirate it with a fine needle. Or you can ask for a painkiller. Ice packs in combination with painkillers are the usual route. A topical antibiotic may also be necessary, which often speeds up healing.

Nipple Infections

Yeast or bacteria can get into the nipple, causing impetigo (a bacterial infection) or thrush (a yeast infection). Either infection can cause symptoms of burning and irritation. Your doctor can usually distinguish which kind of infection you have through your symptoms and will prescribe the appropriate medication. If the infection doesn't clear up, your doctor will culture it to sort out the problem.

Yeast

When yeast occurs in the mouth or nipple, it's called thrush, but it's caused by the same organism involved in vaginal yeast infections. Here, the two organisms usually responsible for this infection are Candida albicans or Monilia. Both organisms like warm, sweet places and can be transferred from the baby's mouth to your nipples. When sore nipples suddenly erupt, thrush is the likely cause. A culture for yeast may confirm thrush, and the baby's mouth should be examined for white patches—classic signs of thrush. It's possible, however, for you to be infected and not the baby.

One of the classic triggers of yeast infections are antibiotics. In fact, if you've been treated for mastitis with antibiotics, you may wind up with thrush a few days later! Diabetics (yeast love sugar) and women with a compromised immune system (due to illness or even HIV) are also classic thrush victims.

To treat thrush, 1 percent miconozole cream is usually prescribed, which must be worked well into the nipple before and after nursing to relieve the burning. If the baby also has thrush, this cream will get into the baby's mouth during nursing, and cure him, too.

If you seem to be continuously plagued by yeast, you may need to adjust your diet. Anemia, for example, is a common cause of chronic yeast infections because it impairs your immune system. Consult your doctor about this.

Chronic Subareolar Abscess

This is an uncommon infection of the sebaceous glands around the nipples. Bacteria is the culprit again, having gotten inside the glands via breastfeeding or lovemaking suckling. The glands get blocked, and your breasts get red and form painful boils. This is an unsettling and ugly sight, but it's quite treatable. The gland needs to be surgically opened, or the infection will keep coming back. Antibiotics and minor breast surgery are the treatments.

Maybe You're Pregnant

If sore nipples suddenly develop after several weeks or months of comfortable breastfeeding, you may be pregnant. As you know, nipple tenderness is often one of the first symptoms of pregnancy, caused not by an irritant, skin infection, or bad latch but by hormonal changes.

In this case, none of the suggestions provided above will be of much use. Some women disregard pregnancy as a possibility because their menstrual cycles haven't returned. As discussed in chapter 10, you can get pregnant during breastfeeding without noticing the resumption of your period. Nipples can also become sore for a day or two during ovulation.

The duration of this nipple soreness is highly individual, but many women report that it often lasts throughout the entire pregnancy, disappearing right after the birth of the new baby. To make matters worse, your milk supply may also decrease. When this is the case, you may not have as much breast milk as before, but you certainly continue to breastfeed until your next baby is born, and even after if you wish. (See chapter 10 for more details.) If you don't want to wean, the following techniques can help you cope with the soreness during this pregnancy.

- Try acetaminophen or use the breathing techniques you learned in your first pregnancy to help manage pain during breastfeeding.
- Try varying your nursing positions more often.
- Ask—if your nursing child is old enough—for her to be more gentle or to nurse for shorter time spans.

(Breastfeeding during pregnancy is discussed more in chapter 10.)

OTHER CULPRITS

There are some other origins of breast pain you should be aware of. Some of these are not exclusive to lactating women.

Cysts

Although a breast lump in a breastfeeding woman is most often a galactocele or lacteal cyst (milk cyst), caused by plugged milk within the ducts, it should be carefully watched. A galactocele, usually very tender, will shrink and disappear within a matter of days.

Until you have the milk cyst diagnosed, however, you may have a bit of a scare. Essentially, you should perform a breast self-examination every month or so and look for any suspicious lumps or changes in your breast during feeding. A milk cyst is simply a self-contained lump in your breast that is filled with milk. Your doctor can easily aspirate the cyst with a long, fine needle.

Some women are plagued with painful cysts that are not related to breastfeeding. If this is the case, the cyst can be drained. If you find a painless lump that is not a cyst, have it biopsied. See your doctor as soon as you discover it.

Cyclical Breast Pain

If your menstrual cycle has returned (see chapter 10), breast and nipple tenderness may be a premenstrual symptom. All of the following symptoms are signs of PMS: swelling, tenderness, and lumpiness (water retention can create a lumpy feeling). Stopping caffeine and taking vitamin E may be helpful in alleviating these symptoms. (Review my book *The Gynecological Sourcebook* for more information on PMS and cyclical breast pain.)

Mastalgia

This simply means "breast pain." This pain can come and go, or else persist. Mastalgia varies from minor irritation a couple of times a month (often a PMS symptom) to debilitating pain. Mastalgia is broken down into cyclical pain—which is the same as hormonal breast pain—noncyclical, chronic pain; and non-breast-origin pain (a pain that has nothing to do with your breasts).

Noncyclical Breast Pain

This is usually anatomical (meaning that something inside the breast itself is causing the pain) rather than hormonal. Cysts are usually the origin. Noncyclical breast pain can also be caused by a bruise. *Very, very rarely* it could indicate cancer (most times, breast cancer is painless). This type of pain should be checked out by your doctor. The cure is either finding the source of the pain and relieving it (aspirating a cyst, for example) or being reassured that you don't have cancer by a negative mammogram (these are 85 percent accurate), shrugging, and taking a pain reliever such as aspirin.

Non-Breast-Origin Pain

This is usually a form of arthritis, called costochondritis. Men get this too, and think they're having a heart attack, while women assume they have breast cancer. You'll need to be treated for arthritic pain to relieve it, which can be pinpointed by any primary-care doctor. A pinched nerve in the neck can also cause breast pain, as well as a type of phlebitis (inflamed vein) in the breast. These cure themselves in time.

SOME PAINFUL CONSEQUENCES

Unfortunately, sore breasts and nipples can lead to poor letdown, which in turn can be triggered by pain, fear, fatigue, stress, or alcohol. Decreased nipple stimulation will also lead to poor letdown, the result of a bad latch, topical anesthetics on the nipple, or nipple shields. The final consequence of poor letdown can be an exacerbation of the problem that caused the soreness to begin with, which caused the poor letdown: more engorgement, which can lead to both a plugged duct or mastitis. All this can affect your baby, who may not get enough milk, as well as your entire milk production, which will gear down.

To avoid this unfortunate chain of events, make sure you investigate the origin of your breast pain and get pain relief—and don't stop breastfeeding. Avoid topical anesthetics, nipple creams, and nipple shields. Follow the guidelines for self-care discussed in earlier sections of this chapter. If you need help with letdown, request an oxytocin nasal spray. Also review the section in chapter 4 on letdown "foreplay."

Medication Musts

If you're prescribed medication for your pain, it's crucial to ask the following:

1. *How will the drug affect my baby?* Doctors will often recommend weaning when prescribing a drug for you, not because the drug has been found to affect the baby but because doctors fear lawsuits. This isn't a good enough reason to wean, though—particularly if the baby is less than six months old. Remember, for almost all medical problems, medications are available that are safe to use during breastfeeding. Safe painkillers include acetaminophen and codeine.

2. *Will temporary weaning harm me or the baby?* Abrupt weaning can be a traumatic experience for both of you, leading to even more pain. In all cases of temporary weaning, replace a nursing with a pumping session (or manual expressing).

3. *What are the treatment options?* Don't settle for a drug that is contraindicated (not advised) during breastfeeding; ask for one that's safe!

4. Review the Food and Drugs section in chapter 2.

ৎ৯

Many of the triggers of soreness during breastfeeding have more to do with your baby's health than your own. If your baby is ill or unexplainably fussy at the breast, this will lead to a breakdown in efficient breast-emptying, leading to many of the conditions discussed in this chapter. The next chapter will, hopefully, answer many of your questions regarding common infant health problems during breastfeeding.

chapter 8

GROWING PAINS: COMMON AND NOT-SO-COMMON INFANT AILMENTS

his chapter reflects interviews with breastfeeding parents and doctors and offers a sampling of information from the pediatric health literature. Included are discussions of either the most common or the most worrisome pediatric health problems (which may *not* be so common) that may affect breastfeeding. What you won't find is a discourse of every pediatric heath problem; it's just not possible to cover the scope of this subject within one chapter. Consider, then, this chapter as a pediatric "starter kit."

Information on symptoms, diagnosis, and treatment for the numerous ailments discussed below are provided along with separate sections on allergies (page 216), common infections (page 222), special-needs babies (page 225), and hospitalization (page 226).

For most of you, the first section is the one to read, as it discusses conditions ranging from colic to slow weight gain. Since many of you are consulting it because you want answers *now*, it has been organized alphabetically, with cross-references included should you need to review other parts of the book more thoroughly.

THE BABY-C'S

Your newborn may experience any one of numerous conditions while you're breastfeeding that may indicate a more serious illness, but often it is just a "welcome to parenthood" condition that clears up as mysteriously as it developed.

Colic

Colic, one of the most misunderstood infant conditions, has been used interchangeably with "fussiness," "crying," and persistent indigestion. The problem is, there is no one definition of colic other than "intense discomfort." Whether this discomfort is physical or emotional is not yet understood, but this discomfort has a different origin for every colicky baby. Colic usually develops around six weeks of age and lasts until three or four months of age. According to one study, only about 12 percent of all cases of colic last beyond six months.

The symptoms of colic are inconsolable crying with no evident cause. When a colicky baby cries, he will experience a sudden spasmodic abdominal cramping (the abdomen will become distended when this happens), and will typically draw up the knees, grunt, and turn red. The entire body tenses, the fists may clench, and a look of agony comes over the face. The crying usually takes the form of a high-pitched scream. While crying, the baby may swallow a lot of air, which only makes things worse.

Occasionally, passing gas can provide some temporary relief, which is why colic has been associated with indigestion. But colic may be a symptom of a more serious problem, which is why it's important to have the baby examined for things like ear infections, diaper rash (which often indicates a food sensitivity), urinary tract infections, anal fissures, hernia, and so on. Colic is the appropriate diagnosis when no other signs of illness are evident.

Colic usually occurs during the late afternoon or evening and can last for hours. But at least it's punctual, occurring at about the same time every day. And it's finite; it does, after several months, go away. Unfortunately, it can be pretty agonizing for both you and the baby.

What Causes Colic?

Colic has been linked to a variety of sources that include allergies (see the allergy section on page 216), overfeeding, underfeeding, too much or too little hindmilk, too much fat, sugar, or protein, and too large or too small a hole in a bottle nipple. Bottle-fed babies will suffer from colic more frequently than will breastfed babies.

Stress and anxiety in the baby's environment are considered to be significant triggers of colic. Stress causes gastrointestinal discomfort in babies just as is it does in adults. Colic is also seen more often in first babies, and rarely in babies of more mature parents—a clue that first-time-parent jitters, common in younger parents, may be a contributing factor. Unfortunately, the more the baby cries, the more jittery the parents get, creating a merry-go-round of discontent for all.

Other triggers for colic are:

✄ Swallowing too much air (which may occur during crying).

✄ Poor latch (see chapter 4).

✄ When a baby is tongue-tied (see chapter 4).

✄ An overactive letdown (see chapter 4).

✄ Cow's milk protein from your food (or protein from other foods) that may be excreted into the breast milk, causing stomach upset in the baby.

✄ Nicotine secreted into the breast milk (only likely if you're smoking while breastfeeding).

What Should You Do?

If you've nailed down the cause, such as poor latch, too much milk (see farther below), and so on, *fix the problem*. If no apparent reason for the colic can be found, then relieving the colic depends on your baby. Sometimes a colicky baby gets more upset when you try to calm her down. Some babies respond to "white noise"—a blow dryer, vacuum cleaner, running water from a shower or faucet, fan, and so on, turned on either before, during, or after feeding. Other soothing noises to colicky babies are loud ticking clocks, classical music, recordings of heartbeats or womb sounds, and even a recording of the baby's own cry (which distracts, interests, and ultimately calms). Some babies calm down with a car ride. Others seem to do better when you hold them, and while they may still cry they are nonetheless calmer. There is, in fact, a "colic-carry" position, where the infant is held with the head slightly higher than the feet and is straddled across your arms and then gently rocked. (Alternatively, the baby can be held facedown across your lap, head supported by one leg and stomach supported by the other, and then rocked, or even bounced.)

When it comes to breastfeeding, it's crucial that you have a good latch and that you find a position for optimum digestion; this usually means sitting up. (See chapter 4 for more information on positioning.)

Can You Treat Colic?

Not really. In the past, medications that combined barbiturates and alcohol were widely peddled, but they are now considered at best useless, and at worst downright harmful. The general rule for treating colic today is to move the baby around with you, "wearing" or carrying her everywhere. Studies show that four hours of extra carrying per day will cut the crying time in half. Eliminating cow's milk or another culprit food from your diet is the second rule, which is particularly recommended if colic comes on four hours after you eat something with cow's milk. (This is discussed more below and in the allergy section on page 216.)

Sometimes a baby glycerine suppository will help an infant pass gas, providing temporary relief. Antispasmodics and antiflatulent medications are sometimes prescribed as well, while chamomile or fennel teas (a few teaspoons only) have also been known to help.

Certain lifestyle adjustments beyond diet can also have an impact in the areas of smoking (if you absolutely cannot stop, then smoke only when your breasts are full to reduce nicotine levels) or stress (if you're anxious, try to work it out).

If you are eliminating cow's milk from your diet however, be sure to read labels: Foods you don't suspect of containing cow's milk often do. If you need to supplement your calcium, do so with nondairy foods combined with calcium supplements (each Tums tablet contains 200 mg—a cheap way of supplementing). You need roughly 1,500 mg a day when you're breastfeeding.

If eliminating cow's milk doesn't help, something else you are eating may be bothering the baby. Common culprits include citrus fruits, broccoli and cauliflower, prunes, wheat, nuts, beef, eggs, or even spicy foods and garlic. You'll need to conduct your own "control" studies and eliminate various foods to see if indeed they seem to have an effect. It will take roughly two to four hours after you've eaten these foods for them to get into your breast milk, after which the baby may be bothered during or after a feeding.

Crying vs. Colic

A baby may cry frequently but not be colicky. Crying is the baby's only way of communicating some unmet need. And no, it's not "good for the baby to cry," or good to "let the baby cry it out." What's good is to respond to the cry the best way you can. So it's important to exhaust all possibilities before you label the baby colicky. Here's the "top ten" list for what a crying baby may be trying to tell you:

1. *I'm hungry.*

2. *I want to suckle* (for comfort).

3. *I want to cuddle.*

4. *I'm tired of this position!*

5. *I'm bored. Do something to relieve the monotony!*

6. *Change my diaper.* (Or, *I don't like this kind of diaper!*)

7. *I don't feel well* (could be a million reasons).

8. *I'm constipated or have gas.*

9. *I can't handle all this stimulation!*

10. *I'm tired or overtired.*

And of course let's not forget: *I want my toy.* It is when the crying turns into a soprano wail or scream that you should begin to suspect that something is very wrong, such as illness or extreme emotional distress.

Cuddling and carrying an upset baby is a tonic whose power must never be underestimated. A 1986 study found that infants of first-time parents who spent more time being held and carried cried less. Younger babies had more dramatic results; three extra hours per day of carrying a one-month-old baby actually reduced the amount of crying time by 45 percent.

Constipation

As discussed in chapter 6 (in the "pees and poops" section, page 156), it's normal for a breastfed baby over four months old to go as long as a week without a bowel movement as long as the stool is soft, the baby's growing well, and everything gets covered in poop when the weekly event occurs. But whenever you notice an absence of regular bowel movements, it's important to note the "signs of good eating" discussed in chapter 6. Feel the baby's abdomen and make sure that the baby isn't in pain. A healthy abdomen should feel soft rather than hard. A hard or distended abdomen is a sign that the baby may be full of gas, which may be contributing to the constipation. The longer the baby goes without a bowel movement, the larger the stool should be. If this isn't the pattern, have the baby's health evaluated by a doctor to rule out more serious conditions such as hypothyroidism (discussed below). You may need to give the baby a suppository or a supplement to get the stools moving again.

Diarrhea

Occasional diarrhea is usually nothing to worry about. In this case, the baby may be reacting to something you've eaten. Persistent or chronic diarrhea is a sign that something's wrong, and is most commonly caused by a reaction to antibiotics, a flu bug or other illness that irritates the stomach lining, or the introduction of solids into the baby's diet. In this case, the diarrhea is labeled "nuisance diarrhea," and it goes away in a few weeks. The general rule is that no matter how loose the stools are, if the baby seems to be healthy otherwise and is not losing weight, you don't need to worry. What's loose for one baby may be normal for another.

If weight loss or dehydration is accompanying the diarrhea, make sure your doctor rules out the following:

- a bladder infection

- food allergies (see the allergy section farther on)

- galactosemia (rare; discussed farther on)

ℬ irritants in your own diet, such as large amounts of fruit, laxatives, and so on

ℬ infant lactose overload (too much breast milk, discussed farther on)

ℬ an intestinal illness or parasite

Treatment

If possible, the underlying health problem triggering the diarrhea must be fixed. In some cases, this may mean weaning, particularly if galactosemia is diagnosed; in other cases, it may mean eliminating certain irritants from your own diet. If the baby becomes dehydrated, a rehydration solution will help, but in most cases, breastfeeding should continue and will eventually help the diarrhea to pass.

Fussiness

Fussiness does not necessarily mean a baby is malnourished or colicky. In fact, all babies usually have fussy times that occur in the late afternoon or evening, but this does not necessarily make them "fussy babies."

If the baby seems to want to eat every hour or so and always seems to be hungry, fussy, and gassy, then this may mean the baby is suffering from infant lactose overload, or "too much milk." This is discussed on page 214 of this chapter.

Fussiness has a lot in common with crying; the origins are often the same, ranging from overtiredness and overstimulation to loneliness and physical discomfort. And like adults, babies simply have different temperaments, which is why one baby will react completely differently in a given situation than another.

Dealing with Fussiness

Once you get to know the fussy pattern of your baby, you'll develop your own tricks for speedily handling the problem. Until this day comes, experiment with the following: burping; a diaper change; dressing or undressing baby; checking for crumbs or hair in a sock or between the toes; bathing baby; massaging baby; rocking baby or putting him in a sling or carrier (studies show that babies who are carried around or "worn" cry less); changing the environment (going from a noisy room to a quiet room or vice versa); going for a walk outside; playing certain music. Then again, none of these suggestions may help! Sometimes the only way over a fussy period or fussy time is to just go through it!

Galactosemia

In this serious condition, the liver enzyme that normally converts galactose to glucose (a simple sugar) is missing. Without it, the baby is unable to metabolize lactose and can suffer from severe symptoms that include vomiting, weight loss, cataracts, and even mental impairment. In fact, any lactose in the baby's system will damage the baby's liver.

Galactosemia is fortunately quite rare, occurring in only 1 in 85,000 births. It develops within the baby's first few weeks of life. In the past, babies with galactosemia did not survive. Today, the treatment for galactosemia is complete weaning, because breast milk is loaded with lactose. The baby is then placed on a lactose-free formula, which is given via bottle. A feeding tube from the breast is not recommended in this case because it may allow some breast milk into the baby's mouth.

Hypoglycemia

Newborn hypoglycemia means that the baby's blood sugar is too low. This situation can occur if you had either a difficult pregnancy, involving perhaps toxemia or gestational diabetes, or a long, difficult delivery. An IV of glucose given to you for any reason during delivery can also trigger newborn hypoglycemia.

In the past, most hospitals simply gave each baby over a certain birth weight glucose water to prevent hypoglycemia, but this makes newborn jaundice worse, unless that glucose water is given by feeding tube at the breast, which will help stimulate breast milk production. Now the standard practice is to check for the condition and treat it only if it's present in the newborn. A glucose level over 30 mg/dl in a full-term baby and over 10 mg/dl in a preterm or low-birth-weight baby is considered normal.

Anything less than that is considered hypoglycemia. The best treatment in this circumstance is to breastfeed the baby as frequently as possible. Unrestricted breastfeeding for at least ten to twelve feedings in the first twenty-four hours will provide the baby with enough fluid and calories for the first couple of days of life.

If the baby's glucose levels remain low, glucose water can be given via feeding tube at the breast, discussed in chapter 6. For very tiny (due to prematurity) or very ill babies, glucose will be given intravenously.

Hypothyroidism

The thyroid gland makes thyroid hormone by extracting iodine from various nutrients. Thyroid hormone drives the metabolism of every cell in your body; without enough thyroid hormone, you cannot function properly and the entire body slows down, causing constipation, extreme fatigue, dry skin, and a variety of general ill-health symptoms. In a baby, thyroid hormone is crucial for proper growth and development. A baby born with either a low-functioning thyroid gland or no thyroid gland is said to have congenital ("present at birth") hypothyroidism. If the baby develops hypothyroidism shortly after birth, it's known as neonatal hypothyroidism. Both are serious conditions that are a major cause of mental retardation in the Third World.

The good news is that in North America all babies are automatically screened at birth for this condition with the "heel pad" test, where blood is taken from the heel and the baby's thyroid function is tested. Only about one in 5,000 babies are born with either low or no thyroid hormone. The treatment is to place the baby on thyroid replacement hormone for life. This amounts to a small pill taken each day that can be crushed and placed into the baby's mouth until solid foods are started.

Occasionally, breastfeeding can mask congenital hypothyroidism because thyroid hormone is secreted into the milk and passed along to the baby. In this case, the baby will benefit from your thyroid hormone as long as you're breastfeeding but will begin to show signs of hypothyroidism as other foods are added to the diet and the proportion of the baby's nutrient intake provided by breast milk begins to drop. (For more information, review my book *The Thyroid Sourcebook*.)

Jaundice

A baby who turns yellow has jaundice. Neonatal jaundice is an extremely common problem that affects roughly 50 percent of all normal, full-term infants within the first week of life. Breastfeeding is usually the best medicine for a jaundiced baby, yet despite this undisputed medical fact, jaundice is still the most common excuse for stopping breastfeeding. In most cases of jaundice, there is absolutely no reason to stop breastfeeding. (Exceptions are discussed farther on.)

What Is Physiological Jaundice?

There are three types of neonatal jaundice, but about 95 percent of all cases take the form of normal jaundice (aka physiological jaundice). When your baby has jaundice, the skin turns yellow because the red blood cells that are being retired from service result in the production of a yellow pigment called bilirubin. Bilirubin builds up faster than the baby's immature liver is able to handle. In essence, neonatal jaundice is caused by too much bilirubin. The good news is that bilirubin simply passes through the baby's stools. The more the baby poops, the faster the bilirubin is eliminated.

So *where* are all these red blood cells coming from? When the baby is still in utero, less oxygen is available to the baby than outside the uterus, when the baby begins to actually breathe air. Therefore, a fetus's body will manufacture more red blood cells in order to have enough oxygen for its brain and heart.

Normally, it's the liver's job to remove blood waste like bilirubin from the body. But in this case, the baby's liver is new and cannot work fast enough to remove the bilirubin. The result is the development of jaundice by the second or third day of life. The jaundice will usually peak between the fifth and seventh day and then begin to recede.

The Symptoms

First, the baby's eyes turn yellow, then the face, followed by the trunk of the body. The last body parts to turn yellow are the fingers, toes, palms, and soles. Unless the baby is breastfeeding often and without any imposed time limits, she will not get enough colostrum to stimulate her bowels. When this happens, the symptoms may be more severe as the levels of bilirubin rise. A jaundiced baby will also be sleepier, and may need to be awakened to breastfeed. (See the section in chapter 4 on sleepy babies, page 116.)

Bilirubin levels that get dangerously high become toxic to healthy cells. Brain cells may be destroyed (and will not grow back), and a condition known as bilirubin encephalopathy, or kernicterus, can result. While today these conditions are rare, they can still occur if the bilirubin isn't excreted.

Treating Physiological Jaundice

Breastfeeding as long as possible and as often as possible is the best treatment. Usually the jaundice will clear up within two to three days of good breastfeeding. You should be seeing dark, greenish brown stools (the green is meconium, backlog waste from intrauterine life), which go to brown as the meconium is cleared. Meconium stools are a sign that the baby's gut is getting cleared out. (Review the "pees and poops" section in chapter 6 for more details.) The baby should not be given any water or glucose supplement unless there's a good medical reason and that supplement is administered via feeding tube at the breast (see chapter 6). That way the baby will still be able to suckle colostrum from the breast. Otherwise, these supplements are not only completely useless in lowering bilirubin levels but fill up the baby and discourage the frequent breastfeeding that can help offset the jaundice. If a supplement is needed and cannot be given by feeding tube at the breast, pumped milk, banked milk, or formula are the best solutions (in that order), not glucose water.

If the jaundice is more severe, a treatment known as phototherapy may be employed. Here the baby is either placed in direct sunlight or put under a special fluorescent light in the blue-to-white range, known as a "bililight." The light actually helps to break down the bilirubin through the skin. The baby is placed under the lights wearing only a diaper, with the eyes covered and protected. If you're rooming in with the baby, bililights can be brought to your room, and you can even breastfeed the baby for brief periods of time during the bililight therapy. If the phototherapy is taking place in the hospital nursery, you can usually be with the baby during the therapy. Bililights can also be rented, so that you can conduct the therapy in your own home. The length of treatment depends on the baby's condition, but it can range from continuous treatment for a long stretch to a period of a few minutes every few hours.

Another form of phototherapy involves a fiberoptic wrap that the baby simply wears around the body. This is considered a better method if the baby needs continuous treatment, and it does not require any eye protection.

Breast-Milk Jaundice (BMJ)

This rarer form of jaundice, clinically termed late-onset jaundice, is thought to be triggered by something in the breast milk itself. In this case, some factor in your milk seems to be interfering with the baby's ability to eliminate the bilirubin. BMJ makes up approximately 2 to 4 percent of all neonatal jaundice cases. Fifteen percent of all siblings of previous BMJ cases will develop it, too. Unfortunately, normal jaundice (the most common, discussed above) is often misdiagnosed as BMJ. In order to have BMJ, the following symptoms must be present:

1. Jaundice begins five to seven days following birth, *after* breast milk has come in.

2. Bilirubin rises rapidly and reaches its peak between day seven and ten.

3. Bilirubin remains elevated, and jaundice remains more or less evident for weeks, sometimes for as long as three to six months.

4. Bilirubin levels drop rapidly when breastfeeding stops and rises again when it's started (although it is not necessary to stop breastfeeding to "test" this.)

5. All pathologic causes of jaundice are ruled out.

To date, no one really knows the cause of BMJ. In most cases, you don't need to stop breastfeeding; it will clear up on its own without any treatment, but the baby will just take longer to eliminate the bilirubin.

If the bilirubin levels are dangerously high, then you may need to stop breastfeeding for a maximum of twenty-four hours (pumping or expressing to keep up your milk supply) and substitute with your own heated milk (see below), donor milk, or formula. Most doctors will tell you to continue breastfeeding while they monitor bilirubin levels in the baby.

Research has found that heating the breast milk at 56°C for roughly fifteen minutes seems to help lower bilirubin levels. Weaning should not be recommended as a treatment for BMJ.

Pathologic Jaundice

This rare form of jaundice occurs when something causes the baby's red blood cells to break down faster than normal, causing bilirubin levels to rise faster and higher than normal. In this case, the baby is either born jaundiced or will develop it within twenty-four hours of birth. Breastfeeding should be continued, and phototherapy may be necessary. In extreme cases, the baby may need a blood-exchange transfusion.

Can You Prevent Physiological Jaundice?

Yes! The earlier and more frequently you breastfeed your newborn, the less likely it is that jaundice will develop. All studies done on preventing jaundice have concluded this. As discussed in chapters 2, 4, and 6, colostrum works like a laxative and helps eliminate bilirubin faster than any other compound.

The other way to prevent jaundice is to avoid supplementing breastfeeding with glucose water or any other liquid—except when medically required, by feeding tube at the breast. Supplements fill up the baby and discourage breastfeeding as frequently as nature intended. Research has shown that glucose water supplements may actually raise bilirubin levels. That's why it's important to put breastfeeding on your birth plan, as discussed in chapter 3.

Nursing Strike

When your baby suddenly refuses to breastfeed, seems perfectly healthy otherwise, and will feed via cup, spoon, or bottle, you are looking at a "nursing strike." And you should take it personally. In this case, your baby is trying to tell you something by refusing your breast. Some reasons why your baby is on strike:

ஐ Hurt feelings. Someone has hurt the baby's feelings. A baby-sitter may have dropped the baby; someone may have yelled at the baby.

❧ A bad experience at the breast. Perhaps the baby bit you accidentally, causing you to scream. Perhaps the smoke detector went off when the baby was in the middle of feeding and you jumped up and scared the baby. There could be a hundred different scenarios causing your baby to associate the breast with something "bad."

❧ A sudden switch to a new schedule. Whether you're weaning, going back to work, or traveling, your baby may have a strong reaction to any changes in the feeding schedule.

❧ Pain that worsens during feeding. If your baby has sore gums from teething or even an ear infection, breastfeeding may be uncomfortable, resulting in a strike.

❧ A more serious illness or infection. A baby suffering from a urinary tract infection, gas, or many of the other conditions discussed in this chapter may suddenly refuse to nurse. However, a nursing strike is more common when the baby is in perfect health.

❧ A change in your milk due to a menstrual period (the baby will want to breastfeed after your period, however) or even pregnancy (see chapter 10).

❧ A reaction to a new deodorant, body powder, lotion, perfume, hair spray, detergent, fabric softener, and so on.

Strike vs. a Desire to Wean

A nursing strike is often confused with a baby's natural tendency to wean. To make the distinction, it's important to note what a nursing strike is characterized by:

1. Abrupt refusal of the breast vs. gradually prolonging intervals between nursing.

2. Clear distress when offered the breast vs. disinterest and nursing just to be "polite."

3. Clear acceptance of breast milk from other feeding tools, such as cup, spoon, or bottle vs. a disinterest in breast milk altogether and a desire for solids.

4. Breast refusal under one year of age vs. a baby older than a year.

Negotiating a Nursing Strike

In order to get your baby back on the breast, first rule out any physical cause for the strike. Check for sore gums, an ear infection, or a urinary tract infection.

If the baby appears to be in perfect health, review the chain of events that most recently preceded this strike. Was someone other than yourself looking after the baby? Do you recall anything unusual when you last breastfed? Whether you can remember anything out of the ordinary or not, apologize profusely and repeatedly to the baby. Talk to the baby when you apologize; many mothers report that their apologies are accepted. As you apologize, cuddle the baby. Then take the baby to bed with you, continuing to cuddle and comfort. Try to get that skin-to-skin contact. This will help make the baby drowsy and comfortable and more ready to accept the breast.

Keep apologizing and keep cuddling. Something has disturbed the baby's universe; order needs to be "restored" in the baby's eyes before breastfeeding can resume.

Nursing strikes should usually resolve in about a day. If the strike continues for longer, take the baby to the doctor for an evaluation. You may need to pump/express your milk until things are back on track.

Refusing One Breast Only

Whenever a baby seems to reject only one breast either right from birth or just out of the blue, take care to rule out a medical condition such as a stuffy nose, an ear infection, a hernia, a misaligned neck vertebra, and so on.

There may be some other reasons for preferring one breast over the other. For example, after an episode of mastitis (see chapter 7), your breast milk may taste saltier from the affected breast.

If this preference starts right at birth and you can't find a reason for it, as long as you don't mind nursing from one breast only, do it. Eventually, your unsuckled breast will return to your prelactating size, and you may look a little lopsided. But if the baby is getting enough milk (see chapter 6) don't worry about it.

Phenylketonuria (PKU)

PKU is an inherited metabolic disorder that leads to mental impairment if left untreated. Here the baby is unable to metabolize the amino acid phenylalanine, present in breast milk, which prevents normal brain and central nervous system development. Because of the severity of PKU, most hospitals in North America routinely perform a heel-pad test for PKU at birth, drawing blood from the baby's heel. If the baby tests positive for PKU, the general rule is to feed the baby some breast milk with a special formula called Lofenalac, which contains no phenylalanine. Keep in mind that there are many false positives for PKU. Have your baby retested for it after six months to confirm any positive diagnosis.

Poor Muscle Tone

If your baby seems to have a floppy "rag doll" posture, there may be low or poor muscle tone. (If the baby arches a lot, this could signal overactive muscle tone and is discussed in chapter 4, page 123.) Both low or overactive muscle tone are signs that the baby's nervous system is temporarily immature or that the baby may even be neurologically impaired. (See the section on special babies farther on.) If you suspect this kind of problem, have your baby's health evaluated.

Slow Weight Gain

First, review the Weight Watching section in chapter 6 before you suspect slow weight gain. The general rule is for babies to at least double their birth weight at about five to six months and triple their weight by one year. In some cases, slow weight gain is hereditary; mothers of slow-gaining infants often discover that they, too, were slow in gaining weight as infants.

It's also important to look at the baby's length and head circumference. For example, a thin baby with a normal length and head circumference may be very healthy but simply have some minor feeding problems.

If a breastfed baby isn't thriving, there are three main questions to ask before the cause of slow weight gain can be identified:

1. *Is the baby feeding well?* Is the latch correct; do you understand the principles involved in good breastfeeding management, and so on?

2. *Are you producing enough milk to meet the baby's needs?* The latch may be perfect, but a baby who isn't getting enough milk will not gain well.

3. *Is the baby healthy?* Poor weight gain despite a good latch and good milk supply may point to an underlying health problem.

If the cause is the baby's feeding, once good breastfeeding has been established, weight gain should follow soon thereafter (review chapter 4). If you're not making enough milk, this could result from any number of things, including poor breastfeeding management (review chapter 5) to pain, stress, diet (caffeine and alcohol affect milk production), medications, or even a health problem such as thyroid disease that interferes with milk production.

Otherwise, the baby's health should be evaluated to rule out a more serious health problem, such as a urinary tract infection, heart problems, hypothyroidism, cystic fibrosis, and so on. Table 8-1 indicates the complex medical history that needs to be taken in the event of slow weight gain. The most difficult factor in dealing with slow weight gain is finding the cause. Once that's found, fixing the problem will result in normal weight gain.

Generally, breastfeeding should not be interfered with or interrupted unless there's a good medical reason. In fact, formula-fed babies tend to become fatter babies, which puts them at risk for not only a variety of other diseases but for obesity later in life, and subsequently at risk for developing obesity-related conditions such as diabetes, high blood pressure, and heart disease.

Spitting Up

While many parents worry that their babies are spitting up too much, this is perfectly normal, even if the baby seems to be spitting up a lot of milk after each nursing. As long as the baby is peeing, pooping, and growing, there is nothing to worry about.

Table 8-1
SLOW GAINING INFANT SPECIAL HISTORY

Mother

Name _____

1. Do you smoke? ____ Which brand? ____ How many per day? ____

2. Any thyroid problems at any time in your life? ____
   Are thyroid medications being taken now? ____ What kind? _____
   Dose? ____ Last time you had your blood tested for thyroid level? _____

3. Coffee? ____ How many cups per day? ____ Caffeinated sodas (colas)? ____
   How many caffeinated sodas per day? ____

4. Are you taking any medications? ____ Birth control pills? ____ Prescription? ____
   Nonprescription? ____ Which vitamins? ____

5. Do you have a busy lifestyle? ____ If so, why (name activities)? _____

6. Alcohol consumption? ____ How much per day? ____ Week? ____ Month? ____

7. When baby breastfeeds, do you feel: Tingling ____ Burning ____ Filling ____ Feeling ____
   Leaking on other side ____ Nothing ____ Other ____

8. Marriage relationship: Good ____ Average ____ Poor ____ Are you seeing a counselor? ____
   Other children? ____ Ages ____ Breastfed? ____ How long? ____

9. Quiet environment for nursing? ____ If not, why? Describe (example: loud music, freeway noise,
   dogs barking) _____

10. Do you have any blood pressure problems? ____

11. Are you in good health? ____ Describe problem _____

12. Do you eat regular meals? ____ How do you rate the kind of food you eat? ____ Good ____
    Poor ____ Excellent ____ Brief diet history _____

13. Any source of anxiety or tension? _____ Describe _____

14. How many children in your family while growing up? ____ What number were you? ____

15. How would you describe your mother when you were little? Busy ____ Warm ____
    Troubled ____ Great housekeeper ____ Distant ____ Nurturing ____ Other ____

16. What advice has she given you about spoiling the baby? _____

Baby

Name _____ Date of birth _____

1. How often is the baby fed in the daytime? _____

2. Breast milk only? ____ Other? ____ Do you feed from each breast at each feeding? ____
   How long on each breast? ____

Table 8-1 continued

3. How long does the baby take to finish a feeding? ____
   Does the baby pause a lot during feeding? ____

4. Who initiates end of feeding? You ____ Baby ____

5. How do you rate the sucking? Poor ____ Weak ____ Strong ____ Average ____
   Don't know ____

6. Number of wet diapers per day? ____ Are paper diapers used? ____

7. Number of stools per day? ____ Per week? ____ Consistency? ____ Color? ____

8. Burping easy? ____ Technique used? ____ When burped? ____ Does he spit up? ____
   Vomit? ____ How often? ____

9. Activity of baby: Active ____ Placid ____ Average ____
   Developmental progress: Average ____ Advanced ____ Slow ____

10. Is a pacifier used? ____ What kind? ____ How much usage? ____
    Does he suck his thumb or fingers? ____

11. Night sleep pattern: Time put to bed ____ Is this on a regular basis? ____
    List awake times _____

12. Baby healthy? ____ Any problems since birth? ____ If so, what? ____ Jaundice? ____
    How high was the bilirubin? ____ Had any medications? ____ If so, what? ____

13. Ever had a urinalysis? ____ When? ____ Any other tests (especially those for slow
    weight gain)? ____ If so, what? _____ Where? _____

Birth History

1. How long were you in labor? _____

2. Were medications given during labor or delivery? ____ If so, what? _____

3. First time the baby was put to breast was ____ hours/minutes after birth.
   Did the baby take to it easily? ____

4. Was it a difficult birth? ____ If so, describe problem _____

5. Home birth? ____ Hospital with rooming-in? ____ Hospital with baby only in nursery? ____
   Were you separated from the baby for any length of time? ____ If so, why? _____
   And how long? ____

6. Any medications taken during pregnancy? ____ If so, what? _____

7. Any medications taken after birth? ____ If so, what? _____

Source: Riordan, Jan. A Practical Guide to Breastfeeding. Boston: Jones and Bartlett Publishers, Inc., 1991: 222–223.

What you might want to know is *why* the baby spits up. The most common reasons are either too strong a letdown (the baby will be choking or gulping hard in this case), which will usually adjust to the baby's needs in time, or a baby's strong gag reflex. But many babies spit up for no reason at all.

Sometimes spitting up indicates an allergy of some kind to a food you or the baby may be eating, or to a medication. This is especially likely if the baby suddenly starts spitting up out of the blue. And, of course, the baby may also be allergic to formula! In fact, spitting up is a common problem with formula-fed babies. Vitamin supplements such as iron or fluoride are also classic triggers of spitting up. If you suspect a more serious problem, have your baby's health evaluated by a doctor. This is also advisable if your baby is regularly spitting up after every feeding or is projectile vomiting. While this is often normal, it can also be a symptom of pyloric stenosis, a condition where the muscular wall of the tube connecting the stomach to the intestines is overdeveloped. In this case, the milk does not pass easily from the baby's stomach into the intestines, resulting in poor nourishment. This is discussed next.

In almost all cases, the baby outgrows spitting up within four to six months. Until spitting up subsides, you can try to be more gentle in handling the baby after a feeding, keeping the baby upright. If you think the spitting is related to too much milk, see the section on too much milk below.

Pyloric Stenosis

This more serious condition indicates a structural problem with the tube that connects the stomach to the intestines. Symptoms of pyloric stenosis usually develop between two to eight weeks of age and are usually more common in firstborn white male babies. Classic symptoms are regular spitting up or even projectile vomiting, when the baby's stomach muscles force the milk up the throat and shoot it out of the mouth. The vomit or spit-up in this case can be shot forward several feet. At first, this type of vomiting may happen only occasionally, but in time it occurs more frequently until you notice it after every feeding.

The treatment for this condition involves a simple surgery called a pyloromyotomy, which repairs the tube. The baby can begin breastfeeding again as soon as six to eight hours afterward, but you may need to limit feedings for a short time.

It is possible for your baby to have projectile vomiting and be perfectly healthy, but when it happens once a day or if your baby isn't growing well, see a doctor to rule out this condition.

Too Much Milk (Infant Lactose Overload)

When the baby is "overdosing" on breast milk, it's called *infant lactose overload*. In this case, you're making more milk than your baby needs or can handle.

The following have been cited as factors that can cause the breasts to overproduce milk:

- Breasts that are oversensitive to the suckling (this may even run in families).

- Increased stimulation due to nursing multiples or too much pumping/expressing milk between feedings (common if you're donating breast milk).

- Certain medications such as domperidone, chlorpromazine, or any other drug that alters dopamine levels.

- Too much caffeine, causing the baby to sleep less and eat more.

When your breasts produce too much milk, the baby is full before even finishing one breast, never getting to the fat-rich hindmilk. The baby winds up getting only the protein-rich foremilk, which digests quickly and leaves the baby unsatisfied. Worse, the foremilk is loaded with lactose, something the friendly bacteria in the baby's intestines thrive on; the more bacteria, the more gas. The result is a hungry, gassy, fussy baby. You'll also notice that the baby is constantly peeing, pooping, and gaining more weight than is normal for that age.

In addition, too much breast milk can increase the risk of plugged ducts, mastitis, and even engorgement (see chapter 7).

What's the Solution?

Make sure the baby finishes one breast, and then simply pump out the other until it's comfortable. Prior to feeding, you can also express a little milk to avoid overfilling the baby. Don't switch breasts midfeeding, and don't offer the second breast until the first breast is *completely* emptied—even if that takes two or more feedings. By doing this, your breasts should eventually make less milk, because they will not be as stimulated. To relieve the baby's gas, give the baby five to fifteen drops of lactase (Lactaid) before you nurse.

In some cases, no matter what you do, your breasts continue to overproduce milk. All you can do in this case is to express the milk and donate it to a milk bank.

ALLERGIES

In an age of questionable air quality and unquestionable chemicals, allergies have become a way of life for millions of parents and children's doctors. The good news is that breastfed babies develop fewer allergies than do formula-fed babies, but they are not completely immune to them. The list of allergic symptoms is long and includes sinus inflammation/hay fever, runny nose, eczema, diarrhea, coughing, asthma, conjunctivitis (pink eye), nausea, vomiting, lack of appetite, and respiratory infections (discussed later). Dark circles under the eyes, called "allergic shiners," are also telltale signs of an allergy.

Maybe It's Something You Ate

Many of the conditions discussed in the previous section are often cited as food allergy "reactions," such as diarrhea or colic. Most food allergy symptoms, however, will suddenly appear after exposing the baby to the substance and then suddenly disappear when the offending substance is removed from the baby's diet. It's also important to realize that two babies allergic to the same food may develop completely different symptoms; for one it may be diarrhea, while for another it may be nausea and vomiting. Furthermore, babies can have reactions to many different foods that belong to a single botanical family. In other words, an allergy to almonds can show up when the baby is exposed to apricots, cherries, nectarines, peaches, plums, or prunes, because all these foods share the same botanical family. (See table 8-2 for a list of food families.)

Table 8-2
FOOD FAMILIES

Common Foods	Relatives
Almond	Apricot, cherry, nectarine, peach, plum, prune
Apple	Crabapple, pear, pectin, quince, rosehips
Asparagus	Chive, garlic, leek, onion, shallot
Avocado	Bay leaf, cinnamon
Banana	Arrowroot, plantain
Basil	Marjoram, mint, oregano, peppermint, rosemary, sage, savory, spearmint, thyme
Beef	Buffalo, butter, cheese, gelatin, goat, lamb, milk, pork, sheep, veal, and all related products
Beet	Beet sugar, chard, spinach
Black pepper	White pepper
Blueberry	Cranberry, huckleberry
Buckwheat	Rhubarb, sorrel
Cabbage	Bok choy, broccoli, Brussels sprouts, cauliflower, Chinese cabbage, collards, horseradish, kale, kohlrabi, mustard, radish, rutabaga, turnip, watercress
Carrot	Anise, caraway, celeriac, celery, coriander, cumin, dill, fennel, papaya, parsley, parsnip
Cashew	Mango, pistachio
Cheese (hard)	Mushrooms, truffles, yeast
Chicken	Cornish hen, duck, pheasant, quail, turkey, and all their eggs
Clove	Allspice, guava
Cocoa	Chocolate, cocoa butter, cola
Coconut	Date, hearts of palm
Codfish	Haddock, pollack, whiting
Cottonseed oil	Okra
Crab	Crayfish, lobster, prawn, shrimp
Currant	Gooseberry

Table 8-2 continued

Common Foods	Relatives
Deer	Elk, moose, reindeer
Gin	Pine nut
Ginger	Cardamom, curry, turmeric
Grape	Brandy, champagne, cream of tartar, raisin, wine, wine vinegar
Lettuce	Artichoke, chamomile, chicory, dandelion, endive, escarole, tarragon, safflower, sesame, sunflower seed, and their oils
Melon	Cantaloupe, casaba, chayote, cucumber, gherkin, honeydew, pumpkin, squash, watermelon
Nutmeg	Mace
Olive	Olive oil
Orange	Grapefruit, kumquat, lemon, lime, tangerine
Oyster	Abalone, clam, mussel, scallop, snail, squid
Peanut	Alfalfa, bean (garbanzo, kidney, lima, navy, pinto, soy, string), bean sprouts, black-eyed pea, carob, guar gum, hydrolyzed vegetable protein, lentil, licorice, pea
Pomegranate	Grenadine
Potato	Pepper (cayenne, chili, red, green), eggplant, paprika, pimiento, tobacco, tomato
Salmon	Trout
Sea bass	Grouper
Sole	Flounder, halibut, plaice, turbot
Sweet potato	Jicama, yam
Tuna	Albacore, bonito, mackerel
Walnut	Butternut, hickory nut, pecan
Wheat	Bamboo shoots, barley, corn, graham flour, millet, molasses, oat, rice, rye, sorghum, sugarcane, wild rice

Source: The Allergy Sourcebook, © *Lowell House, 1995.*

When you're breastfeeding, the baby can be sensitive to a substance in your own diet that's passing through to your breast milk and, if your baby is getting over an upset stomach, sometimes to the milk itself—particularly if the baby is lactose intolerant (discussed next). Vitamins, dyes, or additives can also trigger a reaction. But the most common offender is cow's milk and cow's-milk products. Other popular allergens include chocolate, cola, corn, citrus fruits, egg whites, peas, beans, tomato, wheat, cinnamon, artificial food colors, shellfish, pork, beef, onion, and nuts.

Lactose Intolerance

This is usually a temporary condition in which the baby lacks the enzyme lactase to break down the lactose in milk. It is most common following an upset stomach. Intolerance that is limited to cow's milk while the child thrives with breast milk is NOT considered lactose intolerance, but an allergy to cow's milk. True lactose intolerance means that the baby is unable to tolerate *any* form of lactose, no matter what mammal it comes from. Symptoms of lactose intolerance include bloating and/or diarrhea. Generally, if diarrhea persists, it is best to rule out other causes (see the diarrhea section on page 200) before you accept lactose intolerance as the culprit; this condition has a tendency to be overdiagnosed.

Treatment depends on the severity of the intolerance, but there should be no reason to stop breastfeeding. In the worst-case scenario, you can feed expressed/pumped milk to your baby along with lactose drops. Once the condition clears up, you can continue to breastfeed normally.

As the child gets older, tolerance for such foods as ice cream, cheese, yogurt, and buttermilk may improve, because the lactose in them has been broken down somewhat during processing. You can also give an older child lactase in a pill such as Lactaid.

The Process of Elimination

No matter what the offending food is, the only treatment is elimination of that food from the diet. This has to be done carefully so you can be sure that you've nailed down the culprit. During breastfeeding, most doctors or allergists will suggest keeping a daily chart of both yours and the baby's diet. You must also become an avid label reader to avoid accidentally exposing the baby to the food substance in a by-product. It's a good idea to ask your doctor for a list of related by-products to watch out for. For example, if the baby is allergic to cow's milk, you'll want to avoid the following: casein, caseinate, sodium caseinate, whey, lactose, lactoglobulin, lactalbumin, and curds—all common substances found in countless packaged goods.

If you think that you've successfully eliminated the offending food, you'll need to prove your theory by reintroducing the baby to the product to see if the allergy returns. Keep in mind, too, that it's not uncommon for the baby to outgrow the allergy completely.

What if you can't nail down the culprit through elimination? In this case, you need to look at medications you might be taking or environmental causes for the allergy, such as fumes from new carpets, lead (if the baby is a toddler and licking walls), dyes in stuffed animals the baby is sucking on, pesticides, and so on. This is discussed farther below.

Can You Prevent a Food Allergy?

Many food allergies can be avoided by exclusively breastfeeding at least six months before introducing the baby to solids. By then, the baby's enzyme system is mature enough to metabolize proteins. Furthermore, if you introduce various foods to the baby slowly, you can watch for any reaction with each new food you introduce. Often an immediate dislike for a food indicates a potential allergy.

If it seems as though the baby is reacting badly to almost every new food encountered, *breastfeed longer*. In this case, the baby's enzymes may not be developed enough to handle other foods. In fact, you may need to breastfeed more often as the baby gets older to replace the calories the baby would normally get from solids.

Another way to prevent an allergy is to look at your family history. Forty to 80 percent of all allergies are inherited.

Food Sensitivity vs. Food Allergy

There is a difference. A food sensitivity acts like an allergy but doesn't evoke a response from an allergy test. In this case, the symptoms are more vague and subtle. In fact, a common cause of hyperactivity in children is a sensitivity to food that may be missed in a classic allergy test. Common reactions to food sensitivities also include a fast pulse, fatigue, and migraine headaches (classically triggered by cheese, nuts, or wine). If you suspect a food sensitivity, an elimination diet once again is the treatment.

Something in the Air

Environmental factors are often responsible for a host of baby and child-hood sensitivities and allergies. The laundry list of offenders includes: environmental toxins such as pesticides and chemicals; natural inhalants such as pollens and animal dander; skin irritants such as chemicals in laundry products; lanolin; lotions; dyes; synthetic fabrics; grass; or poison oak or ivy.

Under these circumstances, symptoms may range from skin rashes, hay fever (runny nose, rhinitis, irritated eyes), and asthma to a true allergic reaction called "anaphylaxis," where there is a sudden drop in blood pressure and a swelling of air passages that warrants emergency medical attention. (Anaphylaxis can also be caused by food allergens, particularly nuts.)

In Here or Out There?

If you suspect that something in the air is affecting your baby, you must consider which of two environments may be responsible: the interior or the exterior one. The interior environment is the one you can *control,* and hence eliminate the allergen if possible. This is where you can begin to hunt down culprits such as carpeting, dust mites, secondhand smoke, laundry products, and so on.

There is little, alas, you can do to control the outside environment, except limit your child's exposure to various irritants.

When to See an Allergist

If you've discovered the allergy source yourself and have successfully eliminated the problem, you don't need to seek out a specialist unless the baby's health is in question or the allergy has "mysteriously" returned.

In cases where an environmental agent is suspect (interior or exterior), it's best to have the baby tested to nail down the exact allergen. (Keep in mind that skin tests for allergies don't work on small babies, however.) The problem with airborne allergens is that they're difficult to pinpoint without the aid of allergy tests.

Where do you find an allergist? Ask your family doctor or pediatrician, friends and family members, or anyone else you trust. (In Canada, you'll most likely need a referral.) If you don't like the first allergist you see, get a second opinion. Always make known your preference to continue breast-feeding.

COMMON INFECTIONS

Even with the protective antibodies of colostrum, breastfed babies are not completely immune to the numerous viruses and bacteria they're exposed to on a daily basis. It's all part of life on Earth. Discussed below are the most worrisome infections, but this chapter cannot possibly replace a more thorough pediatric health book. The good news is that if your breastfed baby should fall prey to an infection, it will usually be a less severe one. If your breastfed baby is chronically sick with respiratory infections and flulike symptoms, an allergy may be the cause, rather than a virus.

The Flu

While it's common for everybody in the family *except* the baby to get the flu, breastfed babies can and do submit to it from time to time. When your baby has the flu, a virus is the cause (either a rotavirus or reovirus). The typical symptoms are upset stomach, vomiting, and diarrhea, which will last for a few days and then slowly disappear. Keep breastfeeding. Most babies will breastfeed more often when they're sick. If your baby doesn't want all your milk, simply express what's left to avoid engorgement, and take the baby to the doctor; poor appetite may be a sign of a more severe illness. Once the baby is well again, breastfeeding should resume as though the episode never happened.

Usually a baby with the flu can still digest enough breast milk to bene-fit from its nutrients and fluids before it's spit up. So don't bother with sub-stitute fluids that friends, family, or even some doctors may suggest, such as soda or jello water; these don't work as well as simple breastfeeding. If there's not enough breast milk to satisfy the baby, you'll need to rehydrate the baby with fluids your doctor can prescribe. Review the sections on spitting up and diarrhea in the first half of this chapter.

What Should You Do?

Keep track of the baby's general health, wet diapers, and weight loss. (This is discussed in chapter 6). If you suspect that the baby is dehydrated because of diarrhea and vomiting, give the baby an oral rehydration solution that your doctor recommends; do not use water. Rehydration solution can be given with a spoon, dropper, or cup.

Flulike Symptoms

A baby may appear to have the flu when in fact it's really chicken pox, measles, mumps, or something else. All these viral infections tend to be less severe in children than in adults, but it's important to consult your doctor for advice. Mumps will not affect male children's ability to reproduce unless they have the virus during puberty. Again, follow the flu rules above for breastfeeding.

Upper Respiratory Infections ("Colds")

These infections rank number one when it comes to infant and childhood illness. Again, viruses are the most common cause, but these infections are less common and severe in breastfed babies. Symptoms include a cough and hoarseness (when crying or talking). The best way to clear the cough is to have a cool mist vaporizer in the baby's room at night, which will moisten mucous membranes and loosen the cough. If you don't have a vaporizer, take the baby into the bathroom and run a hot shower to create steam, wrapping the baby up in a large towel. This should produce the same results as the vaporizer.

A baby battling a respiratory infection will have trouble nursing. That's because the baby's nose is stuffed, which makes it harder to breathe. You can try to steam the baby right before nursing, or nurse in a steamy bathroom. Sometimes walking outside in cool, moist air will help, or you can wash the baby's nose with nose drops or breast milk, or aspirate the baby's nose with a nasal aspirator. In an older baby, oral decongestants such as Dimetapp or Triaminic, or a decongestant nose drop given fifteen to twenty minutes prior to a feeding should allow you to breastfeed normally.

Pneumonia

Although this is rare, when pneumonia develops in a breastfed child it is usually less severe. In this case, the baby may be placed on antibiotics as a preventive measure so that a bacterial infection does not develop.

If the baby needs to stay in the hospital and be placed in a tentlike structure that is filled with mist to help clear the infection, there isn't any reason to stop breastfeeding. You can either take the baby out of the tent to feed or climb into the tent with the baby and nurse there.

Meningitis

Meningitis is when the thin membranes that cover the spinal cord and brain, called meninges, become inflamed. This is a serious condition that is fortunately uncommon. In a young child or baby, meningitis is usually less severe than in older children. In fact, it's often associated with other viral diseases such as measles, mumps, or even herpes.

The symptoms, which vary depending upon how mild the meningitis is, can include headache, fever, nausea and vomiting, abdominal pain, rash, and sometimes a stiff neck (more likely in older children).

You must take the baby to the hospital ASAP for treatment, which usually involves a spinal tap and intravenous antibiotic therapy until the cause (viral or bacterial) can be determined. Continuing breastfeeding actually helps to lessen the trauma for the baby.

Herpes

Because herpes is so prevalent in the adult population, it is also seen in babies who are exposed to the virus during childbirth. If a doctor knows that a mother has herpes during pregnancy, a cesarean section is usually performed to prevent exposing the baby to it. Nevertheless, this isn't a foolproof system.

The problem with herpes in babies is that the infection isn't always obvious until a few days or even weeks after birth. Symptoms of herpes can include extreme fussiness, convulsions, and abnormal sleepiness. After that, you will usually see sores on the baby's skin and inside the mouth, which will probably prevent a good latch during breastfeeding.

If You Suspect Herpes

Unless you yourself have herpes, there is no way that your baby has it. If you have a history of herpes but have either not informed your doctor prior to the birth or did not have a cesarean section, be sure to let your doctor know now. If your baby becomes ill, get to the doctor ASAP. This is a serious disease that can be fatal to the baby.

Recently, the FDA approved the use of a new drug specifically developed to treat neonatal herpes. In the meantime, have yourself and your partner screened for herpes. Regardless, it is always a good idea to wash your hands with soap and water before breastfeeding.

SPECIAL BABIES, SPECIAL NEEDS

If your child has Down syndrome or is neurologically impaired, breastfeeding is even more important. In fact, breastfeeding helps protect many of these children from respiratory infections and digestive upsets, ailments that tend to plague special-needs babies more than normal babies. But breastfeeding these babies can present some special challenges.

Neurologically impaired babies fall into two categories: those with overactive muscle tone and those with low muscle tone. There may also be other symptoms such as an arching of the body (feeding an arching baby is discussed in chapter 4); overreaction to stimulation; biting movements, especially when swallowing (called a tonic bite reflex); weak suck, swallowing, and gag reflexes; and nonrhythmic sucking.

Common Breastfeeding Problems

When there's neurological impairment, the nervous system is either immature or physically undeveloped, causing these babies to have a weak suck (see chapter 4) or poor suck-swallow reflex. These babies may also be sleepy babies, which means that you'll need to awaken them to feed. If this is the case, see a lactation consultant or pediatrician so you can fine-tune a technique (some are discussed in chapter 4) that facilitates at least partial breastfeeding. In fact, the stimulation these babies get from the suckling action and skin-to-skin contact is important for their overall development.

Only in severe cases will breastfeeding not be possible. But even then you can still feed the baby your expressed/pumped milk using an alternate feeding tool (see chapter 6).

WHEN THE BABY'S HOSPITALIZED

Sometimes your baby may need to spend time in the hospital. Whether the baby is premature (see chapter 6), has a cardiac problem, or is being treated for severe viral infection, being separated can affect both mother and child emotionally, as well as the breast milk supply. Review chapters 5 and 6 and the letdown section in chapter 4; with good breastfeeding management, the baby's hospitalization doesn't have to interfere with your plans to breastfeed or your plans to feed the baby your breast milk.

In fact, the sicker the baby, the more crucial your milk is. It will not only boost the baby's immune system, preventing more infections that may aggravate the condition, but will also help the baby maintain calories and weight. Studies have also found that when a sick baby has unlimited access to the breast, recovery is more rapid.

"Regression Therapy"

When in the hospital, the baby may regress to behavior you thought was outgrown. This is a normal reaction; the baby instinctively does what is necessary to recover faster. In some cases, the baby may want to nurse more often. In fact, it's not unusual for an ill child who is almost weaned to suddenly revert to breastfeeding several times a day. (Sometimes this behavior is the first sign of an illness.) Or a baby who is exclusively on solid foods may suddenly refuse the foods and want to return to exclusive breastfeeding. Other habits such as thumb-sucking or longing for an outgrown toy are also normal. Once the baby's health returns, he'll just pick up where he left off in terms of development.

The baby may also become needier emotionally—screaming hysterically, for example, if you leave the room for just a short while. This is a normal part of the separation anxiety that occurs when the baby's hospitalized. This should be taken very seriously; do everything you can to be with and comfort the baby. When separation anxiety is ignored, the baby may cope by becoming more detached from you. So, if you get the cold shoulder and find that the baby prefers the hospital staff's company to yours, take this as a sign that the baby is very depressed and in despair. Do everything you can to reestablish a bond with the baby, and if possible, room in by sleeping on a cot in the baby's hospital room.

%ව

While this chapter may be one kind of survival guide, going back to work presents unique challenges that often are not anticipated until you're actually in the workplace. But even if you're not returning to work, if you believe in a woman's right to breastfeed regardless of occupational status, the next chapter should prove something of an eyebrow raiser.

$\mathcal{B}$REASTFEEDING IN THE $\mathcal{W}$ORKPLACE

$\mathcal{J}$ust because you're returning to work doesn't mean you have to stop breastfeeding. There is currently a worldwide effort to create baby-friendly environments in hospitals, communities, and workplaces. Employers are beginning to realize that women with small children are now the fastest-growing segment of the female work force; they're also realizing that by creating an environment that is more open to breastfeeding, fewer absences will result from childhood illnesses or mothers' infections from insufficient breast emptying.

Alas, the baby-friendly workplace doesn't exist for all women, and so this chapter explores how to make breastfeeding work despite a baby-hostile environment and includes suggestions for lobbying your employer for better conditions for breastfeeding mothers. Finally, alternatives are discussed that every working breastfeeder should consider before returning to work.

THE BABY-FRIENDLY WORKPLACE

Companies that adopt baby-friendly policies will not only save money and increase productivity but will actively contribute to *lowering federal deficits and protecting natural resources.*

Women who breastfeed as long as possible will have more protection against breast and ovarian cancer, which will save health-care systems millions of dollars. Encouraging breastfeeding reduces the industrial contaminants released in the manufacture of formula and the materials used to package that formula.

Babies who breastfeed for as long as possible will suffer from fewer ill-nesses, which will reduce health-care costs and significantly reduce absen-teeism, creating a more productive workforce. Finally, since breastfeeding delays ovulation, it acts as a natural contraceptive (albeit not 100 percent ef-fective), helping to create longer gaps between pregnancies, resulting in fewer maternity leaves!

Overexposed

One of the most important challenges for a baby-friendly workplace is to eliminate toxins from the working environment. The easiest toxin to elim-inate is secondhand smoke. Smoke-free workplaces are therefore better places to work in than smoke-filled workplaces.

Chemicals used in the workplace that are classified as hazardous by the appropriate government bodies must be publicized to all employees, detail-ing the relevant components, hazards, and handling instructions specific to that hazard. This enables working mothers to decide whether to stop breastfeeding when they return to work, to stop working to continue breast-feeding, or to find another job in a hazard-free environment. Of course, many hazardous chemicals will have more serious consequences for preg-nant women than for breastfeeding women: and in some cases, those chem-icals may damage future fertility. Tables 9-1, 9-2, 9-3, and 9-4 (on pages 245 to 253) list known hazards to breastfeeding, fertility, and pregnancy, but while they can provide a general guideline to determine whether substances in your workplace will interfere with breastfeeding, they cannot substitute for a discussion of your concerns with your doctor *before* you stop breast-feeding. Keep in mind that all foreign compounds that appear in your blood also appear in your breast milk. Yet toxin exposure is less critical during breastfeeding than it is during pregnancy, especially during the first trimester.

Keep in mind that there is only limited documentation that concerns the symptoms, consequences, or *lack* of consequences of exposing babies to various toxins through breast milk. With the growing demand for this in-formation, however, La Leche League International offers a search service for both toxicological and pharmacological substances and their effects on breastfeeding. In Canada, the Toxicological Index database (Infotox), open to Americans and Canadians, provides peer-reviewed information concerning chemicals identified in the workplace that may appear in breast milk; 5,500 substances are included, of which 2.7 percent have been recognized as being transferred by milk.

Various drug and poison hotlines (listed locally) offer considerable information on toxins affecting breast milk. Specific concerns can also be explored through the NIOSH-TIC database, maintained by the National Institute of Occupational Safety and Health (NIOSH), available on disk at various university and public libraries; NIOSH Information Dissemination can be accessed directly by calling (513) 533-8287. Finally, the Centers for Disease Control (CDC) in Atlanta, Georgia can be consulted at (404) 639-3311.

Is Your Employer Mother-Friendly?

The following human-resources policies are associated with workplaces that are both baby- and mother-friendly as well as human-friendly. Every employee, regardless of sex or parental status, will benefit from the following:

1. *Parental leave policies.* This means maternity-leave benefits ranging from six weeks to six months after the baby is born. Some, none, or all of the leave may be paid by your employer, but the important part of this policy is that you can't be fired or laid off for taking this leave, and that your job is secure when you return.

2. *Flexible working hours.* This can mean a variety of options, including banking time during off-peak hours; tailoring a shift or schedule that works better for you; part-time schedules; job sharing; and longer breaks when necessary.

3. *Affordable infant and child care at or near the workplace.* Often day-care facilities are offered free or at a reduced cost to employees. Some companies even provide transportation to and from the facility, but this is indeed rare.

4. *Adequate breaks during the workday.* Frequent short breaks are perfect for women who need to pump or express milk. For everyone else, they contribute to stress-reduction and greater productivity.

5. *Comfortable, private on-site facilities.* These are private rooms or quarters employees can go to for expressing or pumping breasts; resting due to illness (menstrual cramps, migraines, ulcers); meditation or stress relief; or even stretching during the workday. These facilities need not be luxurious, and can take the form of a "rest room" (what old-fashioned washrooms *used* to have), consisting of a private room *within* a men's or ladies' washroom that has a small cot or comfortable couch, first-aid kits, and so on. Both men and women should have equal access to such facilities.

6. *Tolerance regarding gender, lifestyle preference, and race.* That means no jokes about breastfeeding and pregnancy; no discrimination for any other reason, either.

7. *A clean workplace.* All employees, particularly those who are breastfeeding, have the right to clean washrooms and smoke- and hazard-free environments.

8. *Publicized information regarding employee rights and policies.* All workers should understand their rights regarding leave policies, hazards, and so on.

9. *Access to public-health information.* This includes information on matters such as breastfeeding, nutrition, safe sex, AIDS, and so on. Phone numbers for various organizations (AIDS hotline, or breastfeeding or cancer support groups, for example) are also useful. This information is neither difficult nor costly to assemble and can greatly contribute to health prevention measures, ultimately raising productivity in the workplace.

Price Waterhouse is one example of what a mother-friendly (or baby-friendly) workplace can provide. It has partnered with Sanvita, a division of Medela (which manufactures breastfeeding equipment and supplies) to provide a full, free, breastfeeding program to all employees who are nursing. The program provides employees with a thirty-minute prenatal education phone call with a professional lactation consultant during the last trimester of pregnancy; six weekly outreach telephone calls from a lactation consultant beginning three to five days after birth; as well as unlimited calls to a lactation consultant during maternity leave and during the first four months after returning to work. That's not all. The company will subsidize the cost of the breast pump offered to program participants, and many Price Waterhouse locations may begin offering "mothers' rooms" designed for mothers who need a private place to express or pump. Kinda makes you *want* to become an accountant!

Making Breastfeeding Work

If you're in favor of some or all of the policies above but your current workplace is still stuck in the 1950s, you may be able to help change your workplace to create some friendlier policies that all of your coworkers can enjoy. Many companies actively solicit employee suggestions regarding these matters through open forums, suggestion boxes, and questionnaires. Here are some other ways you can solicit change:

1. Start a group or network of current and former breastfeeders in your own workplace. Together, draft a proposal for friendlier employee policies and submit it to your employer. Include sections in the proposal that *clearly* outline the benefits to employers of friendlier policies, such as less absenteeism, greater productivity, and so on.

2. There are laws in place to protect you from discrimination as a result of pregnancy or breastfeeding. Make sure your employer is aware of the legislation in place to protect you. See the appendix for organizations you can contact to get a copy of existing legislation.

3. Write an article for your employee newsletter about what constitutes a mother- and baby-friendly workplace. Or circulate a memo about your concerns to all employees.

4. Create alliances with international labor federations, and use breastfeeding rights as an entry point for campaigns on human rights, gender equity, and child survival.

5. Alert occupational health workers to the importance of breast-feeding.

Breastfeeding Policies and Legislation

The World Health Organization's Baby-Friendly Initiative has helped to implement baby-friendly policies for women working all over the world. These policies help to prolong exclusive breastfeeding for at least six months. Reports from Finland, Nigeria, the Philippines, and Chile show that WHO's initiative is working; breastfeeding duration rates in the work-place are beginning to catch up to those of stay-at-home mothers. In Israel, more working women breastfeed than do women at home, demonstrating that it is possible for women to work and breastfeed. Working women in North America, however, lag far behind in terms of breastfeeding duration compared with women in other countries and to stay-at-home North American mothers. As a result, Congresswoman Carolyn Maloney of New York is now spearheading a breastfeeding bill in the U.S. Congress, known as the New Mothers' Breastfeeding Promotion and Protection Act of 1998 (introduced in the House). Some of the major perks of this bill propose women be granted "nursing mothers' breaks" (unpaid breaks of an hour per day for pumping milk for a full year after returning to work from maternity leave). The hour can be divided up into two thirty-minute breaks or three twenty-minute breaks. For work shifts longer or shorter than eight hours, "proportional adjustments" will be made. The bill also proposes that a per-formance standard for breast pumps be set so that these devices can be in-spected under Section 513 of the federal Food, Drug, and Cosmetic Act. Employers would also receive tax breaks for setting up lactation stations.

In Canada, a woman in British Columbia made Canadian legal history in 1997 when she won the right to breastfeed at work. A human rights tri-bunal ruled that employers must give breastfeeding employees the time and opportunity to nurse at their desks or elsewhere. In Canada, this is the first ruling stating that refusal to accommodate breastfeeding constitutes dis-crimination on the basis of sex.

Breastfeeding policies and legislation are nothing new. The first policy that recognized the need for breast-emptying was written in 1919 by the

International Labor Organization in the United States when it established the Maternity Protection Convention for working women, which specified two half-hour nursing breaks per day. Many U.S. states and Canadian provinces that adopted similar maternity legislation in the 1920s amended these provisions in the 1950s and 1960s. The ideal situation is a day-care close enough to the workplace so that the mother may visit the baby to nurse.

Unless provisions are made to allow for breast emptying, a breastfeeding mother may suffer from a reduced milk supply (raising pediatric health-care costs) or from infections such as mastitis (causing absenteeism).

Outside of North America, WHO also advocates access to safe drinking water and nutritious food. In North America, this translates into water coolers with filtered water and on-premises restaurants or cafeterias to help breastfeeding mothers maintain adequate nutrition for breastfeeding.

BEHIND CLOSED DOORS

Back on planet Earth, the baby-friendly workplace is often more of a dream than a reality for the average working breastfeeder. So in order to continue to breastfeed when you return to work, you may need to be flexible, open minded, and creative.

One of the chief problems in maintaining breastfeeding in the workplace is the lack of privacy for emptying your breasts (via pumping or expressing) during working hours. Only a fraction of breastfeeding mothers returning to work have the luxury of a private office with a real door that closes. Most women in the corporate sector work in open areas or cubicles, or else in smaller offices with cramped quarters. Many other workplaces don't even provide a desk, as store clerks, nurses, teachers, carpenters, and so forth know so well.

In an ideal world, the best places for public breastfeeding or expressing/pumping would be out in the open, where meals are normally eaten and not excreted! Unfortunately, public acceptance of breastfeeding just isn't what it should be. Use your judgment. If you feel comfortable breastfeeding or expressing/pumping in an open area, do it! This will help raise public awareness and acceptance of breastfeeding as a normal and natural way to feed a baby. But if you feel you need more privacy in your workplace, there are several ways to have it:

1. Use the ladies' washroom, and a portable-style pump instead of a large electric pump. Many women prefer to pump over a sink in case of leaking, while others make do in a private stall. To maximize your privacy, scout out various washrooms in the building and try to time your breaks so they're staggered with everyone else's. If you're lucky enough to have access to a private washroom (gas-station style—you know the kind), you can run water to mask the sound of the pump if you're shy.

2. Go into a stairwell. Drape a blanket or tablecloth under a staircase to make a tent area for pumping. In many large high-rises, you'll find that stairwells are hardly ever used.

3. Find an isolated storage area or storage room. Make a deal with a custodian or janitor to use one of *their* areas.

4. If there's a restaurant or coffee shop near your office, use its facilities during off-hours (not during the lunch rush) to express or pump. You may be able to work out some sort of deal with the owner or manager.

5. Use your car. You can cover the windows with sun blinds or blankets and pump or express right there.

LET'S MAKE A DEAL

If you cannot find a way to create the private space you need, one solution is to make a deal with a coworker who does have a private office. If possible, choose someone with whom you have a good relationship. There are a number of ways to ask for the privacy:

1. Swap political favors. "If you allow me to borrow your office at lunch and during one break each day, I'll cover for you when . . ." or "I'll go to bat for you on . . ."

2. Offer to carpool that coworker to and from work once or twice a week so that person can save some money on gas.

3. Offer home-computing services (word processing, printing, Internet access, and so on) in exchange for that privacy.

4. Offer something personal or unusual that that coworker may want. Think in terms of hobbies, crafts, or gardening: home-grown vegetables or fruits; homemade jams; baskets; quilts; paintings or photography; artsy jewelry; needlepoint; knitted items—you get the idea. Deliver goods in exchange for that privacy. One woman who had a birthday cake business gave free cakes to her coworker in exchange; another woman who lived in the country and kept bees sweetened the deal with home-raised honey.

5. Do you have a flair for something you could market? Are you a closet makeup artist, interior designer, wardrobe consultant, clotheshorse (pay that coworker in hand-me-downs!), or business writer (offer to ghostwrite speeches, proposals, resumés)?

6. If all else fails, offer to compensate that coworker financially for the time you'll be using the office. If the price seems too high, move on to another alternative.

When to Empty Your Breasts

Every woman will have a different schedule for breast emptying, but the general rule is to substitute a breast-emptying session (pumping or manual expression) for each nursing you're missing. (See chapter 5 for more details.)

Some mothers begin to pump/express their milk prior to returning to work in order to begin building up a reserve supply of milk that can be fed to their baby by a caregiver when they're out of the house. Other women only begin pumping/expressing when they actually return to work. It's a good idea to have a practice session prior to that return so you can work out the kinks in terms of equipment, timing, and so on. It's also a good idea to pump an ounce or two of milk after the baby nurses in the morning or at night, so you can add to your reserve supply while you're away from home.

How Many Times a Day Should I Pump?

It depends on how long you're away from home and how often you nurse your baby. If you're exclusively breastfeeding, it's best not to go more than three hours without a breast-emptying session. In a typical nine-to-five schedule, assuming you fed your baby at, say, 7 A.M., you would empty at 10 A.M., at 1 P.M., and finally at 4 P.M., assuming you were home in time for supper. If you're working late, you would at least have more privacy in a washroom or private office to empty your breasts. If you are leaving a very young baby who has been nursing more often, you may need to pump or express your milk more frequently to avoid engorgement.

Many women find that their breast milk adjusts to their working schedule, and so eventually they need to pump only once or twice or day, and then breastfeed more frequently when they are at home.

Eliminating the Clues

If you don't want anyone to know that you're emptying your breasts at work, depending on where you're pumping, play music from a portable sound system or radio to mask the sound of an electric pump. If you're in a washroom, you can run water or flush the toilet a few times while you're pumping.

If your breasts begin leaking at the wrong times, you can shut off your letdown by applying firm pressure directly on the nipple for a couple of minutes. To do it discreetly, cross your arms. Your breasts will adjust to your new schedule in a few days, and the leaking should stop.

Finally, wear pump-friendly outfits to work—separate tops, patterns that can conceal leaking stains, and extras stored away in case of an accident. Wearing breast pads will also help.

Stashing the Evidence

Expressed breast milk can be left out at room temperature for at least ten hours prior to refrigerating. Keep the milk in a clean plastic or glass container in your bottom drawer. If your office has a fridge, simply store the milk there. Label the container with your name and a date so others don't mistake it for their own. Many women simply bring a cooler with a couple of freezer packs to work and keep the milk there. (Storing human milk is discussed in detail in chapter 5.)

WHAT DO I TELL THE BABY-SITTER?

For most women, returning to work means the baby will be under the care of a stranger—a nanny, baby-sitter, or day-care worker. Whether you plan to feed your baby from a reserve supply of your own breast milk or whether you're switching to formula (if you've decided to wean—see below), you may find that your baby refuses to take a bottle. In this case, a supplement from a cup, spoon, or other tool can be offered as a temporary measure (see chapter 6 for more details).

Allow your baby to become acquainted with the caregiver before you return to work. In fact, allow the caregiver to practice feeding the baby during this get-acquainted visit, so that the baby can learn to accept nourishment from this new person. Fully brief the caregiver on storage of human milk as well (if you're expressing your milk), discussed in detail in chapter 5.

If Baby Is Bottle Shy

If the baby is reluctant to take the bottle, here are some tips for the caregiver:

- Offer the bottle before the baby is hungry. The baby will greet the bottle with more curiosity and may begin to explore it at this point. A baby who is hungry may become frustrated by the bottle, having been expecting the breast.

- Bring the bottle to the baby after "dressing" the baby in some of Mom's clothing (blouse, bathrobe, scarf, and so on).

- Lay the bottle down near the baby and let the baby take the initiative in finding the nipple.

- Warm the bottle nipple before giving it to the baby by running it under warm water.

- Experiment with different types of bottle nipples. The baby may prefer one over another.

- Experiment with different feeding positions. The baby may be objecting to the position rather than the bottle. (Sometimes resistance may result if the position too closely replicates the one favored for breastfeeding.) Often just moving rhythmically (rocking, walking, swaying) during feeding may do the trick.

ૠ Try inserting the bottle nipple into the sleeping baby's mouth. This may make the bottle seem more familiar to the baby upon awakening.

Balancing Breast and Bottle

Because your baby is taking a bottle from a caregiver when you're absent, you will want to breastfeed as much as possible when you're home. In fact, most babies will have no problem breastfeeding full-time on weekends or when you're home. As long as you're pumping or expressing, your milk production will remain the same. And by breastfeeding full-time when you're home, you can eliminate the need to pump during off-hours. Nipple confusion (see chapter 4) only occurs if the baby is younger than three months. In fact, after six weeks of good breastfeeding, most babies don't have a problem adjusting from the bottle to the breast.

What may happen, however, is a slight increase in milk production on Monday from the breastfeeding you did over the weekend. This may result in more leaking and more pumping or expressing. You'll notice that the pattern of milk production will dwindle again by Friday, then return on Monday. This is a normal process that will rectify itself as you and the baby adjust to your new schedule.

Do keep in mind that a baby who's been separated from you on a regular basis may want to breastfeed more often at night and in the wee hours of the morning to compensate for your absence. This is perfectly normal and nothing to worry about. Sometimes this pattern contributes to a sleepy baby during the day and a very awake baby at night. The result will be fewer feedings during the day, and so you may be able to almost keep up with the baby's needs when you're home without much expressing. Of course, while this pattern is fine for the baby, it may not be fine for you—particularly if you need your sleep. To get more sleep at night, bring the baby into your (non-water)bed at night, or bring the baby's crib into your room. As an alternative, you can move into your baby's room and sleep on a mattress or cot so you don't have to get up to breastfeed as frequently.

WEANING AND IN-BETWEENING

Once you've got the hang of breastfeeding, weaning is a fairly idiot-proof process. If you understand the supply-and-demand concept of breastfeeding (see chapters 1, 4, and 5), weaning is a process that comes very naturally: The more you breastfeed, the more milk you make; the less you breastfeed, the less milk you make. The issues associated with weaning, then, have more to do with balancing the social pressure to wean and your particular feelings about weaning. There is also the very real issue of engorgement, which usually accompanies the weaning process. (Relieving engorgement is discussed in chapter 7, page 178.)

Breastfeeding Sabotage

If you're feeling pressure to wean but aren't ready yet, examine the source of that pressure. As stated in chapter 2, older friends or relatives who never breastfed are often expert at breastfeeding sabotage—uncalled-for comments or remarks disguised as concern but calibrated to hurt you. Often there's an underlying guilt behind the comment, as in, "I never breastfed my kids and they turned out just fine!" Here are some other classics:

1. *The baby looks so thin; maybe you should give her a bottle.* In this case, try retorting with: "She's actually the perfect size for her age. In fact, by giving her a bottle, she'd lose more weight than if I continued to breastfeed!" (Such gratuitous comments rarely refer to a truly thin baby, but if you're concerned about weight, see chapter 8, page 210, on slow weight gain and chapter 6, page 156, on weight watching.)

2. *The baby is far too fat for his age; you should consider weaning him.* In this case, retort with: "He's actually the perfect size for his age. My doctor says he'll gain more weight if I give him formula!"

3. *Don't tell me you're still breastfeeding!* Retort with "Yup! I'm following the recommendations of the World Health Organization. Besides, given our family's history of [breast cancer, ovarian cancer, various childhood illness, etc.], breastfeeding is the best protection!"

4. *If you weaned, your baby wouldn't be so spoiled* [or clingy, or whatever].

Retort with "Gee, Mary's baby was formula-fed, and he's exactly the same as mine."

5. This often comes from a peer, about someone else, but it's intended to rattle YOU. *I can't believe that Helen hasn't weaned Adam yet. My child was weaned and on solids by six months!* Politely reply: "Weaning is such an individual decision. I'd rather breastfeed longer like Helen and follow the World Health Organization's guidelines. That way I know I've gone 100 percent in protecting the baby's health and mine."

Of course, one of the best ways to put any "saboteur" in his or her place is to simply say: "But breastfeeding is so good for me and the baby. Don't you want us to be healthy and well?" That should put an end to the discussion.

When You Want to Wean

The return to work often coincides with weaning prematurely—especially if the baby is at least six months old. Premature weaning is when you decide to wean before the baby does. Otherwise, natural "baby-led" weaning will occur anywhere from three to five years of age.

Mother-led weaning generally begins by eliminating the midday feeding, allowing more comfort during working hours. Prior to weaning, however, it's important to consider the following:

- *Age.* If the baby is six months or older, exclusive breastfeeding can be replaced with some breast milk and some other liquids. If the baby is under six months, exclusive breastfeeding is still more desirable. Also keep in mind that only rarely are babies under a year old ready to wean by themselves.

- *Baby's feelings.* A baby with a strong desire to breastfeed may not be ready to wean. You should distinguish, however, between something that is a habit for the baby and true physical and emotional need.

- *Your feelings.* If it doesn't "feel" right, it probably isn't.

If your child is older than nine months, often just substituting the baby's normal nursing time with an activity or a bottle works. Changing the baby's routine slightly may also help you wean, but the routine for the baby will change anyway once you return to work.

If, despite distractions, routine changes, and substitutions the baby still wants to breastfeed, this is probably a strong hint that the baby simply isn't ready to wean. In this case, the emotional and physical needs your breastfeeding provides cannot be substituted that easily. Depending on the baby's age (discuss this with your doctor), a pacifier or bottle may just do the trick—particularly if comfort is the main motive behind the baby's desire to breastfeed. Nighttime feeding is usually the last feeding to be eliminated, since many babies require that feeding to fall asleep.

If you're combining some breastfeeding with some formula, you'll still be making enough milk to satisfy the baby's need. There is no "right" or "wrong" way to wean, however. Every woman will have different needs and feelings about the right schedule for her. What is important is to trust your own body and to make sure that you know how to relieve the discomfort associated with engorgement (see chapter 7).

SUPERMOM SYNDROME

In one study, 60 percent of working mothers who breastfed admitted to feeling overloaded, regardless of marital status. (Of course, any working mother would probably suffer from the same symptoms, too!) Fatigue and stress, as discussed in earlier chapters, can not only interfere with milk production but with your family relationships as well. If you're having difficulty balancing mothering, working, and all your other roles outside of work, here are some suggestions:

1. Nurse 'n' snooze. Set your alarm thirty minutes earlier and nurse the baby while you snooze. That way you'll have more time in the morning to get dressed and ready for work, and the baby will be fed and content. Try setting your alarm for at least twenty minutes before you have to get up. You can also nurse the baby again just before you leave.

2. Ask your caregiver to stay about half an hour longer when you arrive home so you can just relax with the baby, playing quietly, nursing, or snuggling. During this time, the caregiver can make dinner or quickly tidy up so you don't have as much to do. If your child is in day care, try to have your partner play the "caregiver" role instead.

3. Nurse the baby as soon as you get home. Prolactin will make you feel better and help to relax you, while the baby will feel satisfied early in the evening.

4. Take the baby to bed with you so you won't have to get up for night-time nursing.

5. Take care of yourself. Eat well. Drink lots of water. Exercise. Avoid the bad stuff (caffeine, alcohol, smoking). Go to bed early and nap before dinner if you need to.

Explore Your Options

If you want to return to work while your baby is young, make sure you've explored other options too. For example, consider delaying your return to work as long as possible. Leaving a baby under six months old is always more difficult than leaving an older baby. The older your baby is when you go to work, the easier it will be to combine working and breastfeeding. Explore the option of returning to work gradually (part-time for a few weeks, working your way back to full time). Explore the possibility of job-sharing with another mother in a similar situation. Explore the possibility of "telecommuting"—working at your job from home at least some days a week. This is particularly feasible if you work at a computer all day long. With a modem, you can do everything you need to do from home. Explore whether you can bring your baby to work (particularly if the baby is very young). This is often a solution for women who run their own business. If your partner's income can sustain your family's financial load, have you considered *not* going back to work? This is an ideal solution if your income serves mainly to pay for day care or caregiving. (For more on this topic, check out the book *What's a Smart Woman Like You Doing at Home?*)

Table 9–1
SOME CHEMICAL HAZARDS THAT MAY AFFECT REPRODUCTIVE HEALTH

Hazard	Workers at Risk	Potential Reproductive Effect	Protective Measures
Anesthetic Gases (including halothane, nitrous oxide, methoxyflurane)	Health-care workers in hospitals and dental clinics, veterinary surgeons and assistants, researchers in animal laboratories	*Male workers*: sperm abnormalities; wives/female partners of exposed male workers may experience an increased evidence of miscarriages, premature deliveries, and offspring with birth defects; *female workers*: same as wives/female partners of male workers; *the fetus*: birth defects	Install scavenger units to collect stray gases; monitor air in operating theatre to ensure low levels
Benzene	Workers producing or using solvents, plastics, rubbers, glues, dyes, detergents, paints, petroleum, and other products containing this substance	*Male and female workers*: chromosome changes, linked with leukemia and genetic effects in offspring; *female workers*: prolonged menstrual bleeding and post-partum hemmorhage after chronic exposure; *the fetus*: birth defects, higher incidence of leukemia, illness from contaminated breast milk	Substitute nontoxic or less toxic products; take regular workplace air samples; ensure proper ventilation and safe engineering processes
Beryllium	Ceramic makers, electronics workers, jewelry makers, laboratory workers, nuclear technologists	*Female workers*: pregnancy may exacerbate symptoms of beryllium poisoning and cause death; *the fetus*: may cross placenta and affect fetal development	Monitor workplace levels regularly; install proper ventilation and dust collection devices in the work environment
Carbon Disulfide	Degreasers, glue makers, paint removers, rubber makers, rayon viscoe makers	*Male workers*: decreased libido, impotence, sperm abnormalities; *female workers*: irregular menstrual cycle, decreased fertility, frequent miscarriages; *the fetus*: higher incidence of miscarriage	Monitor workplace levels and reduce to minimum; ensure that prolonged worker exposure is prohibited

Table 9-1 continued

Hazard	Workers at Risk	Potential Reproductive Effect	Protective Measures
Hormones (including androgens, estrogens, progestogens, and synthetic products such as DES)	Workers involved in the extraction, manufacture, and use of hormones, including pharmaceutical workers, laboratory workers, farmers, and veterinarians	*Male workers*: sexual impotence, breast enlargement, infertility; *female workers*: irregular menstruation, infertility, ovarian cysts, breast lumps, cancer of the reproductive system; *the fetus*: may develop enlarged breasts and other signs of sexual maturity as well as abnormalities of the skeletal system, heart, and windpipe; DES may cause cancer in female offspring, genital and sperm abnormalities in male offspring	Monitor regularly to ensure low levels of airborne hormones; isolate the process through engineering design
Lead	Auto manufacturers, ceramic and pottery makers, electronics workers, farmers, pesticide makers, paint makers and users, and typographers	*Male workers*: decreased libido, decreased sperm count, atrophy of the testes; wives/female partners demonstrate adverse effects such as infertility, menstrual disorders, miscarriages; *female workers*: infertility, miscarriages, stillbirths, menstrual disorders; *the fetus*: higher incidence of miscarriages, stillbirths, neonatal death; mental retardation can occur; newborns can be affected by contaminated breast milk	Sample workplace air frequently; provide adequate ventilation; clean work areas regularly
Mercury	Battery makers, ceramic workers, commercial fishermen, dental workers, farm workers, jewelry makers, lithographers, pesticide makers, photographic chemical makers and users	*Male workers*: reduced fertility; *female workers*: miscarriages, stillbirths; *the fetus*: linked with severe brain damage, mental retardation, increased rate of miscarriages and stillbirths	Regular air monitoring and good ventilation; enclose mercury processes; check frequently for spills and vapor leaks

Table 9-1 continued

Hazard	Workers at Risk	Potential Reproductive Effect	Protective Measures
Pesticides (including carbaryl, dibromochloropropane, kepone, malathion 2,4,5-T)	Agricultural workers, commercial and household gardeners, pesticide manufacturers	*Male workers*: chromosomal changes, impotence, loss of libido, decreased sperm counts, atrophy of the testes; *female workers*: miscarriages, chromosomal changes; *the fetus*: miscarriages, birth deformities	Design processes to prevent worker contact with substance; monitor air levels in workplace and keep to a minimum
Vinyl Chloride	Workers involved in the production of vinyl chloride and polyvinyl chloride and its related products	*Male workers*: genetic damage of the sperm, leading to adverse pregnancy outcome in wives/female partners; *female workers*: genetic damage to ovum, miscarriages, stillbirths; *the fetus*: higher incidence of miscarriage, fetal death and birth defects; may develop cancer after exposure during pregnancy	Monitor workplace regularly; use proper ventilation and safe design to keep levels at a minimum

Source: *The Canadian Advisory Council on the Status of Women, Ottawa, 1982.*

Table 9–2

SOME BIOLOGICAL HAZARDS THAT MAY AFFECT REPRODUCTIVE HEALTH

Hazard	Workers at Risk	Potential Reproductive Effect	Protective Measures
Brucellosis (Undulant fever)	Animal breeders, farmers, health-care workers, meat handlers, veterinarians	*Male and female workers:* brueallae may lodge in reproductive organs, leading to local inflammations and infertility; *the fetus:* miscarriage, developmental defects	Control infection in animals; use caution in handling diseased animals and their products as well as the urine and feces of infected humans
Chicken Pox (Varicella)	Day-care workers, pediatric nurses, teachers, laboratory workers, parents	*The fetus:* prematurity, retardation, muscular, skeletal, and heart defects, increased incidence of neonatal death	Isolate infectious person and handle contaminated articles using aseptic techniques; pregnant women should avoid exposure
Cytomegalovirus	Blood-bank workers, health care workers, dental workers, laboratory workers	*The fetus:* infection leading to jaundice, enlarged spleen and liver, heart, eye, and central nervous system damage in the newborn	Use care in handling sputum, urine, semen, blood, and other secretions of the human body; pregnant women should avoid exposure
Hepatitis (Infectious and Serum)	Blood-unit workers, kidney dialysis technicians, laundry workers, laboratory workers, sterilization unit workers	*The fetus:* infection leading to miscarriage, prematurity, stillbirth, and jaundice; enlarged spleen, increased death rate in newborns	Isolate infectious individuals; label potentially infectious specimens visibly; use disposable needles, syringes, lancets where possible; pregnant women should avoid exposure
Herpes Virus Hominus	Health care workers, hospital staff, laboratory workers, research scientists	*Male and female workers:* transmissible genital infections; *the fetus:* fetal death, miscarriage, liver and eye diseases, central nervous system damage	Isolate infected persons or specimens; use caution in handling infected objects

Table 9-2 continued

Hazard	Workers at Risk	Potential Reproductive Effect	Protective Measures
Mumps (Infectious Parotitis)	Childcare workers, hospital staff, laboratory workers, restaurant workers, teachers, parents	*Male and female workers*: inflammation of testes and ovaries, leading to infertility or sterility; *the fetus*: miscarriages, stillbirths, developmental defects, hydrocephalus	Isolate infectious persons, handle specimens with care; alert all workers potentially in contact; promote immunization
Rubella (German Measles)	Childcare workers, hospital personnel, laboratory staff, restaurant workers, teachers, parents	*The fetus*: placental infection may lead to severe congenital abnormalities including deafness, blindness, heart defects, mental retardation	Promote immunization; isolate infected person; handle contaminated material with care; pregnant women must avoid exposure
Syphilis	Blood-unit workers, health care workers, laboratory workers	*Male and female workers*: secondary lesions in organs of the body including reproductive organs, infertility or sterility; *the fetus*: embryal death, infection leading to liver and spleen enlargement, developmental defects	Avoid contact with infected lesions; exercise caution in handling infected equipment
Tuberculosis	Dairy farm workers, health care workers, laboratory workers, laundry workers	*Male and female workers*: tubercular infection of the reproductive organs; *the fetus*: can be infected through blood transfer from the mother or by aspiration of amniotic fluid	Promote immunization; test animals regularly; handle infected specimens with caution

Source: The Canadian Advisory Council on the Status of Women, Ottawa, 1982.

Table 9-3
SOME PHYSICAL HAZARDS THAT MAY AFFECT HEALTH

Hazard	Workers at Risk	Potential Reproductive Effect	Protective Measures
Ionizing Radiation	Atomic radiation workers, dental and chiropractor office workers, hospital employees, scientists	*Male and female workers*: sterility; premature aging of the sex cells, altered genetic material; *the fetus*: damage resulting in prenatal death, mental retardation, birth defects, increased incidence of leukemia and other cancers	Reduce workplace levels to a minimum; use proper shielding techniques; monitor individual exposures using film badge dosimeters and other mobile measuring devices; leave contaminated workclothes at the worksite; maintain exposure records for workers
Noise and Vibration	Assembly line workers, airline attendants, construction workers, garment and textile workers, machinists, motor vehicle drivers, pneumatic drill operators	*Male workers*: sexual dysfunction and decreased fertility; *female workers*: disturbances of the menstrual cycle, increased rate of premature births and complications during labor; *the fetus*: disturbances of uterine circulation in the mother may lead to miscarriage, low birth weight, perinatal mortality	Design machines to ensure minimal noise and vibration; use proper preventive maintenance for equipment; isolate noise using noise absorbing partitions; use sound and sound and vibration absorbing material in floors, walls, and ceilings; install mufflers on all motorized equipment, provide frequent rest periods and job rotations to decrease worker exposure
Nonionizing Radiation	Flight attendants and pilots, food-service workers, health-care workers, radio navigation and radar communication workers	*Male workers*: degeneration of the testes, decreased libido, lower sperm count and motility, abnormally shaped sperm; *female workers*: changes in menstrual cycles, decreased lactation in nursing mothers; *the fetus*: miscarriage, retarded fetal development, congenital defects such as club foot and Down's syndrome	Shield or isolate operations using non-ionizing radiation; check sources regularly for production of x-rays
Temperature (Heat)	Workers in bakeries, canneries, foundries, garment and textile factories, laundries, mines, smelters	*Male workers*: decreased sperm count, atrophy of the testes; *female workers*: decreased fertility; *the fetus*: increased embryal death, low birth weight	Provide adequate training and acclimation, properly designed clothing, and frequent rest periods; enclose heat producing operations as much as possible; ventilate the work area

Source: The Canadian Advisory Council on the Status of Women, Ottawa, 1982.

Table 9-4

Chemcial Hazards that Affect Breastfeeding Mothers

Chemical	Comments
Antimony	Infants of mothers working in an antimony metallurgy plant did not gain weight as rapidly as did infants of unexposed women.
Arsenic	Arsenic can accumulate in a breastfed infant; the infant's blood level should be checked if there is reason to suspect exposure, whether occupational or from sources such as groundwater wells.
Bromide	Bromide, used in photographic laboratories, is a sedative. With maternal intake of 5.4 g/day of bromide, the baby may show bromide rash, weakness, and absence of cry.
Carbon disulfide; tetrachloroethylene	Women working in dry-cleaning plants, viscose rayon plants, photographic laboratories, and chemical industries where proper precautions are not taken have been found to absorb tetrachloroethylene and carbon disulfide. Tetrachloroethylene, used in dry-cleaning, caused obstructive jaundice in a breastfed baby whose mother lunched daily with her husband, a dry cleaner, and had 10 ppm in her milk one hour after exposure. Carbon disulfide, which is a neurovascular and cardiovascular toxin used in the viscose rayon industry, can be found on the hands and clothing of exposed mothers; breast milk levels of 22–306 ug/L were found after commercial exposure, with 16–17 ug/L found in infants' urine. In general, organic solvents should be avoided while breastfeeding. In case of inadvertent exposure, most solvents clear the mother's body within a few days; the time at which breastfeeding can be resumed can usually be calculated from available data.
Chlorinated hydrocarbons	Chlorinated hydrocarbons, many of which are used as pesticides, appear in breast milk because they are stored in body fat. As body fat is mobilized to support breastfeeding, the chlorinated hyrdrocarbons are mobilized as well. In general, the baby receives the greatest dose in utero. Adult body fat has about thirty times the concentration found in breast milk. In the general population, the levels of pesticides in human milk are less than those found in cow's milk. Breastfeeding mothers who work with chlorinated hydrocarbons and suffer acute accidental exposures at work should request advice from their physicians about whether or not to temporarily discontinue breastfeeding and, if so, for how long. Such advice should be based on the half-life and the estimated dose of the chlorinated hydrocarbon involved. Tests are unlikely to be useful, as the results usually take too long to come back; depending on the half-life, the chlorinated hydrocarbon may be cleared from the mother's body by the time test results are available. If testing is indicated, the test of choice is usually the level in (maternal) expired air.

Table 9–4 continued

Chemical	Comments
Dioxins	Dioxins, the best known of which is Agent Orange (used in Vietnam), are found in breast milk from women in the general population. Dioxins are powerful teratogens, but at levels found in the general population, there is no evidence of risk to the infant, and it is recommended that breastfeeding be continued. For massive exposure, a mother should seek advice from her physician.
Estrogen	Estrogen-containing (but not progestin-only) contraceptives may diminish milk supply.
Lead	Lead intake is associated with neurotoxicity in the infant. Older references state that breastfeeding is contraindicated if maternal serum lead is over 40 ug/dL. It should be noted that breast milk may well not be the cause of lead poisoning in a breastfed infant, as lead transfers poorly into breast milk, with a milk/plasma ratio decreasing from 0.1 perinatally to 0.02 from four months on. Children ingest lead from dust, lead-based paint on toys or on paint chips, water from lead-soldered plumbing, or from workclothes worn at a lead-related job. Historically, extremely high occupational exposure of infants to PCBs via breast milk has been associated with lack of endurance, hypotonia, and sullen expressionless facial appearance. Such heavy chronic exposure to PCBs, found in exposed women in the past, is a contraindication to breastfeeding, but should not occur today. In cases of uncertainty or high risk, levels in plasma and breast milk can be measured.
Malathion	The allowable level for malathion in cow's milk is 500 ppb. Studies of the breast milk of mothers living in an area that had been sprayed with malathion for three months found no detectable malathion, with a detection limit of <5 ppb.
Methyl mercury; mercury	Mercury exposure exerts more toxicity prenatally than via breast milk. Exposure via breast milk may affect neurodevelopment in the infant. The set of "safe" levels of total mercury in breast milk is 4 ug/L or less, which would likely be associated with maternal blood levels of 20 ug/L or less.
Nitrate	Nitrate is concentrated in the mother's saliva but not in her breast milk; high levels (as are found in infants fed formula made with high-nitrate water, usually taken from contaminated groundwater wells) can cause methemoglobinemia.

Table 9–4 continued

Chemical	Comments
Polybrominated biphenyls (PBBs); Polychlorinated biphenyls (PCBS)	In the United States, the greatest risk of high exposure to PCBs and PBBs occurs in women who have eaten at least weekly fish caught in contaminated waters, or who are workers who handle PBB/PCBs. PCBs constitute a lifetime body burden, which are transferred less prenatally than by breastfeeding. PCBs are cleared into the fat of breast milk, reducing the burden of the mother and increasing the burden of the infant. Studies of Michigan children, some breastfed by mothers who ingested PBB-contaminated foods, found no effect on physical health and growth, but did show decreased performance of the McCarthy scales of children's abilities and increased body-fat levels of PBBs. Children who are deficient in iron, calcium, zinc, and ascorbate more readily absorb and/or retain dietary lead.
Radioactive materials	Radioactive materials, such as radioactive iodine, gallium citrate, and technetium, may require *temporary* discontinuation of breastfeeding. A breastfeeding mother requiring treatment or diagnosis with radioactive materials should consult with her physician for advice on how long to pump and discard milk, after which she can resume breastfeeding as usual. If the dose of radioactive materials is unknown, so that the appropriate time to resume breastfeeding cannot be calculated, the milk can be tested for radioactivity.
Strontium	Strontium (strontium 89 and 90) appears in breast milk. However, cow's milk has six times as much as human milk.

Source: BC Health and Disease Surveillance *3, no. 2, (February 7, 1994): 20–21.*

chapter 10

$\mathcal{S}$EX AND THE $\mathcal{B}$REASTFEEDING $\mathcal{W}$OMAN

So far, the focus of this book has been on the relationship between you and your baby. This final chapter focuses on another important relationship that breastfeeding affects: the sexual one between yourself and your partner. How does breastfeeding affect your sex life, your fertility, your contraceptive choices, and even another pregnancy? This chapter covers all these issues, including breastfeeding straight through another pregnancy, and breastfeeding children of different ages, or tandem nursing.

WHEN YOU WANT TO MAKE LOVE, NOT MILK

Your sex life changes after the birth of a baby regardless of whether you're breastfeeding or not. The origins of this change lie principally in a change in *lifestyle*. Because you're more fatigued, it may take time before your prepregnancy libido returns. As you may have noticed by now, looking after a newborn involves twenty-four-hour shifts, with little or no sleep. Suddenly there's this connection to your baby that creates an overwhelming sense of communion and caring, a feeling for which many women are unprepared.

As discussed in chapter 1, prolactin, the "mothering hormone," actually creates an emotional feeling of "mothering" that is quite physical. As a result, this feeling can consume your emotional psyche, leaving little or no room for sexual desire. Some women compare the mother-newborn bond to falling in love; everyone else in your life gets "dropped" as you become preoccupied and even obsessed with your baby's welfare. If this description sounds familiar, you're right on schedule. Every mother goes through this; every new father must learn to adjust. A little honesty, sensitivity, and communication goes a long way.

Many experts interpret this mother-newborn connection as an evolutionary device that helps protect the human race. In other words, your feelings for the baby are a biological trait designed to maximize the chances of the baby surviving. Any decrease in sexual desire acts as a natural contraceptive that contributes to better child spacing, while women who may experience no decrease in libido will benefit from a natural period of "lactational amenorrhea" (LAM), or "no menstrual cycle when you're exclusively breastfeeding," which generally lasts at least six months.

While breastfeeding does play its part as a contraceptive, it is not 100 percent reliable; many women who thought so have the children to prove it. If you're experiencing a decrease in libido, chances are it will return to normal once you begin menstruating again. Estrogen levels will increase when your ovulation cycle returns, which will contribute to vaginal lubrication during intercourse. Androgen levels (small amounts of male hormone all women secrete) will also begin to rise when you resume ovulation, which will engage your libido. But there are many other lifestyle and social factors that can affect your libido that have nothing to do with ovulation.

Your Postpartum Physique

Childbirth practitioners advise that even with a normal vaginal delivery, intercourse should be avoided for about four to six weeks, since your cervix is wide open at this point and vulnerable to bacteria. Moreover, if you had a cesarean section or episiotomy, you *must* heal properly to avoid extreme pain or ripped stitches. Until intercourse resumes between you and your partner, the two of you can manually or orally stimulate each other.

When you begin having intercourse again, it will not be the same as it was prior to the pregnancy. First, prolactin, which inhibits estrogen, will not only reduce your libido but may interfere with vaginal lubrication. In fact, dryness is one of the most common symptoms during menopause due to estrogen loss. This means that you may need to use saliva or a synthetic lubricant for greater comfort during intercourse. You may also need to adjust your positions to accommodate a sore perineal area. Lying on top of your partner or using a side-entry position are options worth considering, because they allow you to insert the penis at your own speed.

A drastic change in your postpartum physique may be caused by a very stretched out vagina. Childbirth does stretch the vagina; it never returns to its nice, taut, prepregnant tension. This may dramatically change the sensation for you and your partner, as the grip will not be as tight as it once was.

Don't despair, however. Kegel exercises (contracting the muscle that starts and stops your urinary stream) and abdominal exercises will help to tighten things up, as well as improve your body image. Some of these exercises may not be possible until your stitches from various procedures have healed, but many women report excellent results and are able to regain their grip quite nicely.

If you're having difficulty with grip and "internal belly dancing," to simulate a tighter vagina, sex counselors suggest what I call the "grip trick." This involves getting into a "hands-free" intercourse position and manually closing your vaginal lips around the base of the penis during thrusting. This will improve matters tremendously. As frustrating as your new vagina may feel to you, please don't *ever* consider surgery to "snug it up" unless there's a very good medical reason.

Go with the Flow

Some breastfeeding women may find that their milk lets down during orgasm and sometimes during foreplay (particularly if your partner is stimulating your breasts). Careful planning should take care of this problem—if in fact it *is* a problem. Either make love after a feeding or express or pump your breasts prior to lovemaking. Of course, many men enjoy and accept the letdown as a natural part of things. Attitudes range from fascination with the letdown to actually tasting the milk. You and your partner must simply make the necessary adjustments that meet your level of comfort and discretion. It may help to apply firm pressure with a towel to "shut off" letdown. (Shutting off letdown is discussed in chapter 4.)

A Word about Breastfeeding Arousal

As you may know or may have heard, you can get sexually aroused when you breastfeed. Nursing releases oxytocin, the hormone that causes both letdown and uterine contractions. Oxytocin is also released during orgasm. Don't be embarrassed by this or feel as though you're a sexual deviant. Many women feel the need to masturbate (or have sex with their partners) after nursing. Many women are also aroused by the stimulation of their nipple—which is, after all, a sexual organ, too. Finally, breastfeeding may make you feel fabulously feminine and maternal, which many women find a turn-on. The worst thing you can do is deny yourself these feelings. Pregnancy, childbearing, and feeding are all *sexual* processes that may wake up every sexual impulse within you. In fact, the arousal women feel from breastfeeding may be *why* breastfeeding was unpopular in the more conservative and "retentive" years of the 1950s and 1960s.

Many women also report that they feel a heightened sense of sexual responsiveness when they're breastfeeding. The "mothering" feelings seem to take over in bed as well, creating a deeper bond with their partners.

MILK AND EGGS

A key factor in your sex life while you're breastfeeding has to do with your fertility. How long does it take for your ovulation cycle to return? That depends on how exclusively you're breastfeeding. In cultures where women exclusively breastfeed for at least a year, children are naturally spaced two or three years apart. If this is true, what do we say to women who assumed breastfeeding canceled out ovulation and became pregnant only a few months after the birth of their last child? As more research into the contraceptive effects of breastfeeding continue, the mystery is beginning to unravel.

On the LAM

Lactational amenorrhea (LAM) is considered to be an effective form of natural birth control if you had your baby less than six months ago, have not experienced any vaginal bleeding after your fifty-sixth postpartum day, and you're exclusively (or almost exclusively) breastfeeding, in that you're nursing more than every four hours by day and every six hours by night. Research shows that LAM is 98 to 99 percent effective in women who meet these criteria. Once you supplement the baby with other liquids or solids, however, or skip nursings without replacing them with a pumping/expressing session (which may happen once the baby begins to sleep longer through the night), LAM no longer offers this level of protection, and a backup method of birth control is recommended. In addition, if your baby is not latched on properly, LAM will also not be reliable.

The 2 percent failure rate of LAM accounts for the fact that no contraceptive method is 100 percent reliable. Individual differences in ovulation patterns do occur, and sometimes, even if she is a model LAM candidate, a woman may still get pregnant.

The Period Question

For the majority of you, the contraceptive effect of breastfeeding is directly related to how exclusively you're breastfeeding. Therefore, your periods will return faster if you:

- have a poor latch;
- supplement your breastfeeding with formula or other liquids;
- miss nursings for any reason;
- wean your baby partially prior to six months.

This explains why some women who breastfeed remain infertile for only a few months, while others remain infertile for more than two years.

Women in North America who are not ideal LAM candidates can usually expect their periods to return as early as three months after childbirth to as late as twelve months after childbirth. The addition of solids, bottles of juice, or formula supplements to the baby's diet will bring your periods back faster. In addition, as the baby matures and begins to sleep for longer stretches at night, the contraceptive effects of breastfeeding will further diminish. In one study, researchers found that going six hours or more between feedings and nursing fewer than five times per day were associated with the return of fertility.

When nursing is unrestricted, far more time will pass before the period returns. Sheila Kippley, in her book *Breastfeeding and Natural Child Spacing,* reports that women who practiced total, unrestricted breastfeeding did not see their periods return until an average of 14.6 months after childbirth.

Your own body chemistry has something to do with fertility, too. For example, in the same way that the menstrual cycle varies in terms of days and flow for each woman, so does your body's ability to "bounce back" after childbirth. In other words, women who do nurse exclusively often see their periods return within six months anyway, while women who supplement feedings and partially wean can sometimes wait two years between pregnancies.

Ovulation without Periods

Often ovulation resumes without your knowledge, as is the case with "silent ovulation." Here, a follicle (what an egg is called in its first stage of development) develops from your ovary but never undergoes the physiological and hormonal changes that turn it into an egg. The normal levels of estrogen necessary to build up a uterine lining never occur, while similar levels of progesterone necessary to sustain a pregnancy don't occur either. The result is that you ovulate without ever experiencing a period or a pregnancy.

In other cases, you can get pregnant during your first postpartum ovulation—and also never experience a period. Since ovulation occurs midcycle and menstruation at the end of your cycle, if you get pregnant during your first postpartum ovulation, you will not get your period. In fact, according to a 1982 study in Chile, roughly 2 in 100 women get pregnant within six months of childbirth without experiencing a period.

The Warning Period

The reverse can also occur. You can get a period but not be ovulating yet. This is often the case with the first menstrual period after childbirth, which has been dubbed the "warning period." Here, low, "leftover" levels of estrogen and progesterone (from pregnancy) have caused the uterine lining to build up and shed but have not yet caused your pituitary gland to release

FSH (follicle-stimulating hormone), the sex hormone that signals your ovary to spit out a follicle. After such a "warning period," you'll need to practice contraception unless you don't mind getting pregnant again; this is a sign that the fertility goddess is about to visit you. But don't count on a "warning period"—you might not get one.

When Infertility Persists

Sometimes even some suckling is enough to prevent ovulation. In this case, if your child is older than two and you want to get pregnant again, you may need to completely wean your baby before your cycle returns. It's also possible, however, to experience what's known as secondary infertility. Women who had no trouble getting pregnant with their first child can be plagued by infertility when trying for their second. The causes of secondary infertility range from age (the older you are, the less likely you are to get pregnant) to conditions that often manifest after a first pregnancy, such as pelvic infections that can inflame your fallopian tubes (caused by bacteria entering the cervix during or after childbirth or by various STDs), endometriosis, or male-factor problems. If you're not menstruating, however, this is indeed a hormonal problem that warrants a fertility investigation. If you're menstruating but are still unable to conceive, you and your partner should undergo a full fertility workup with an appropriate specialist. (For more details on infertility, consult my book *The Fertility Sourcebook*.)

Can You Stop Your Periods?

Yes. If your baby begins suckling on your breasts for longer periods of time, your ovulation cycle may become inhibited again. In fact, while your periods may return, they may be irregular until you've stopped breastfeeding altogether. Sudden increases in breastfeeding can occur if your baby is ill and nurses more frequently (discussed in chapter 8), or if you're donating breast milk to a friend and are nursing as well as expressing milk.

Will Periods Affect Milk Supply?

Not only can prolactin inhibit estrogen levels, estrogen can inhibit prolactin levels, causing a slight reduction in milk supply during menstruation. Once your period is over, however, the milk supply bounces right back.

CONTRACEPTION DURING BREASTFEEDING

Abstinence is the only 100 percent way of preventing pregnancy. As discussed above, even if you're exclusively breastfeeding, do not assume that pregnancy is completely preventable unless you don't mind getting pregnant again. Childbirth practitioners recommend spacing your children at least two years apart to give your body a chance to recover from the previous pregnancy. If you're breastfeeding exclusively, it's usually safe to assume at least one to two months of freedom from pregnancy, since it takes at least six weeks for ovulation to resume when you're *not* breastfeeding.

Fortunately, many contraceptive methods are available to breastfeeding women. The only contraceptive that is out of bounds is the combination oral contraceptive (OC) pill. The combination OC, although containing low doses of estrogen, can nonetheless cause changes in the quantity and composition of your milk. As discussed above and in chapter 1, estrogen inhibits prolactin, and vice versa. There is also a risk that the estrogen excreted through your milk could have negative effects on the baby. But you can still take hormonal contraceptives in the form of *progesterone-only* preparations, which can be taken orally, implanted subdermally (under the skin), or injected. Progestin (a synthetic form of progesterone) used alone is also effective because it alters the consistency of your cervical mucus, making it thicker, and causes the lining of your uterus to thin out, thereby discouraging an embryo to implant. Ovulation is also suppressed when the progestin is used for several months.

Of course, barrier methods—diaphragms and gel, cervical caps or sponges, and male and female condoms (the latter not available in Canada) with foam—are always safe and effective.

If you don't want any more children, you may be an excellent candidate for tubal ligation, also known as permanent contraception; similarly, your partner may be a candidate for a vasectomy. Discuss these options with your doctor.

Progesterone-Only Contraceptives

The most popular form of progesterone-only contraception is the "mini-pill," an OC that has progesterone but not estrogen. Since 1991, however, progesterone-only contraceptives have also been available in North America in a subdermal (under the skin) form, called Norplant, and an injectable form, called Depo-Provera. Norplant and Depo-Provera may be more reliable because they eliminate human error. Currently, Norplant is considered to be comparable with sterilization in terms of effectiveness. In addition, progesterone-only contraception is safe not just for breastfeeders but for women who smoke or have other risk factors that prevent them from taking estrogen.

To use Norplant, your doctor inserts six silicone rubber matchstick-size capsules that contain the same progesterone compound used in both the minipill and the combination OC. The capsules are inserted under the skin of your upper arm. Once in place, they steadily release a low dose of hormone into the bloodstream to prevent pregnancy. Norplant, which can be inserted six weeks after delivery, does not interfere with breastfeeding. If your periods have returned, Norplant should be inserted either during your period or no later than the seventh day of your menstrual cycle. Norplant is effective within twenty-four hours after insertion, and the one insertion keeps working for three to five years, depending on which system you've opted for.

Each Norplant capsule is about one-tenth of an inch in diameter, and just under one and a half inches long. It holds 36 mg of the synthetic progestin levonorgestrel, in the form of powdered crystals. The permeable tubes are made of Silastic, a silicone material through which the hormone seeps into the bloodstream, initially at a rate of about 85 µg a day. The amount declines gradually to about 50 µg by nine months, 35 by eighteen months, and about 30 µg at the end of five years. In comparison, the minipill releases about 75 µg of levonorgestrel a day. When the capsules are removed, fertility is restored five to fourteen days later. No side effects have been reported in children conceived after Norplant removal. (Although the product is still too new for this data to be compiled.)

Depo-Provera, which the FDA approved in October 1992, is an injection that works exactly the same way as Norplant, as a "time release" progesterone. One injection of Depo-Provera in the muscle of the arm or buttocks protects you against pregnancy for three months. The active ingredient in Depo-Provera is, again, a synthetic progestin hormone. Both Norplant and Depo-Provera are considered 99 percent effective in preventing pregnancy. To get started with Depo-Provera, you'll need to wait about six weeks after delivery, but it may take at least ten months off Depo-Provera before you can conceive again.

What Are the Side Effects?

The most common side effect of progesterone-only contraception is menstrual-cycle irregularity and irregular bleeding. The bleeding irregularities result from the continuous hormone release and the subsequent thinning of the endometrium. Basically, when there's no thickened lining to be shed, no shedding takes place. With combination OCs, on the other hand, estrogen and progesterone are taken for three weeks and withdrawn for one week, causing *regular* bleeding.

Using Norplant as an example, over a five-year period of use, about 45 percent of Norplant users will have irregular periods, and another 45 percent will have normal periods. The remaining 10 percent will have long stretches of time (three to four months) with no bleeding. Usually, the number of days of menstruation increases, while the flow decreases. In the first year, about 70 percent of users will experience changes in their menstrual cycle. If you're on Depo-Provera, it's common not to have any periods at all, but once you go off, your menstrual cycle returns.

The usual pattern is to have irregular periods in the first year on progesterone contraception, with regular periods developing with longer use. So if you're using this form of contraception, chart your periods; if you go longer than six months without one, ask your doctor if you should continue using this form of contraception.

Other side effects reported include headaches, nervousness, depression, nausea, dizziness, skin rash, acne, change of appetite, breast tenderness (which probably won't happen as long as you're breastfeeding), weight gain, ovarian cysts, and excessive growth of body or facial hair. Breast discharge (in nonlactating women), vaginal discharge, inflammation of the cervix, abdominal discomfort, and muscle and skeletal pain are also reported.

It's important to note, however, that many of these latter side effects are also common *general* complaints, and have not yet been linked specifically to progesterone, as the irregular bleeding has. The most common reason why women discontinue progesterone contraception in the nonlactating population is because of irregular bleeding. But if you're lactating, this shouldn't be a problem, and any bleeding would be very light. Keep in mind that more women have difficulty with combination OCs than progesterone-only forms.

Barrier Methods

If you're planning to employ a barrier method, use condoms without spermicide until six weeks after delivery. Spermicide can enter a dilated cervix and cause irritation. Then you can graduate to a barrier method such as a diaphragm, cervical cap, or vaginal sponge.

Diaphragm

If you already have a diaphragm, put it away now! *You need to be refitted for a new diaphragm following childbirth.* For those of you who have never used a diaphragm, it's a dome-shaped cup with a flexible rim that fits over your cervix and rests behind your pubic bone. It looks like a tiny rubber flying saucer. Inserted before intercourse with spermicide, it blocks the sperm from entering the uterus through the cervix. The failure rate ranges between 10 percent to 20 percent. This is considerably higher than hormonal methods, but much of the failure has to do with improper use and insertion. Diaphragms come in different sizes and styles. You'll need to be fitted for one by either your family doctor or gynecologist. Once you're fitted, you'll be given a prescription, and you can purchase the diaphragm at any drugstore. Then you'll need to go back to your doctor and be shown how to use it yourself. Sometimes you'll need a plastic inserter, sometimes you won't. Go home and practice and see your doctor one more time before you use it, to determine that you're putting it in correctly. Before recommending a diaphragm, your doctor most probably will perform a pelvic exam to make sure that you don't have any physical abnormalities that would prevent you from using one in the first place. It's important to get a diaphragm that fits well; if it's too small, it will expose the cervix, if it's too big, it will buckle. *Get refitted if you've gained or lost more than five pounds, had pelvic surgery, or had another child or abortion or miscarriage.*

Your diaphragm shouldn't interfere with normal activities. Urination or bowel movements shouldn't be affected, and you should be able to bathe and shower normally. If it is interfering with these activities, it may not be in properly or could be the wrong size.

Cervical Caps

Like diaphragms, cervical caps must be refitted after childbirth. The cervical cap is a small, thimble-shaped cap that blocks only the cervix and not the entire upper part of the vaginal canal the way a diaphragm does. The cervical cap thus serves as a "minidiaphragm" with a tall dome. Simply insert the cap with your forefinger and place it over the cervix yourself. About 6 percent of cervical-cap candidates will not be able to find one that fits (shorter or longer cervices are a problem, apparently).

Bad Ideas

If you value your future fertility and general health, stay away from IUDs (intrauterine devices). IUDs are the second-highest cause of pelvic infections, something to which the postpartum woman is vulnerable anyway. IUDs are also associated with secondary infertility, and can cause heavier cramping and flow during your periods. If you *really* want to use an IUD at this stage, discuss the risks with your doctor and be sure you're making an informed decision.

You should also practice safe sex (i.e., wear a condom) if you're not in a monogamous relationship. In addition to AIDS, you can contract a range of STDs that could affect your future fertility. Either the male or female condom (approved as of 1993) will protect you from STDs.

(For more detailed information on these contraceptive methods, consult my book *The Gynecological Sourcebook*.)

BREASTFEEDING DURING PREGNANCY

If you get pregnant while you're still breastfeeding, there's no real reason to stop breastfeeding unless you want to or are experiencing physical complications (discussed below) that warrant weaning. In this situation, many women feel torn between what they think they *should* do and what actually feels right to them. While in North American society, continuing to breastfeed during another pregnancy isn't seen very much, it's a common practice in most countries, particularly developing nations. Often the best decision is not to decide and to simply follow your intuition. For example, you may breastfeed for part of the pregnancy and then wean in a later trimester. In fact, sometimes your baby will begin to self-wean at some point in the second trimester, because the taste and consistency of the milk changes. In addition, hormonal changes will probably affect your milk supply. Estrogen, which normally inhibits prolactin, is released at high levels during pregnancy and may cause a cutback in milk production.

Nutrition Matters

If you're planning to breastfeed during your pregnancy, good nutrition is important for all three of you: your nursing baby, your developing baby, and yourself. The best plan is to see a nutritionist and work out a realistic menu that suits your lifestyle and cultural cuisine. Even if your baby is over a year old, as long as you're eating well you shouldn't have any difficulty nourishing the child outside your womb and the child within. Adequate rest and gaining the right amount of weight are also important factors to consider. For example, if you're eating well but seem to be losing weight throughout the pregnancy, this is a concern. Sometimes consuming extra calories —above the recommended intake during pregnancy—is necessary. In addition, you may need to take extra vitamin supplements. Other times, weaning may be necessary if you can't seem to keep your weight or energy up.

Contraction Action

Because you're still breastfeeding, you will probably experience more uterine contractions than do pregnant women who are not breastfeeding. Nipple stimulation will still trigger oxytocin, which will continue to cause your uterus to contract, regardless of how pregnant you are. Generally this is not a problem, even though it sounds like one. Remember that uterine contractions also occur during sexual activity, which most couples continue during pregnancy too.

If you have a history of premature or false labor, make sure you inform your doctor that you are still breastfeeding. In this case, contractions caused by breastfeeding may interfere with your pregnancy. Moreover, uterine cramping or bleeding is a signal that something's wrong and warrants medical attention. In this case, you may have to stop breastfeeding until after the birth of your new baby.

Feeling Pregnant, Feeding Pregnant

Breastfeeding during pregnancy may be more difficult if you're really *feeling* pregnant! The range of pregnancy symptoms women experience, from nausea to back pain, may make you rethink your weaning decision. In fact, breastfeeding can aggravate certain pregnancy symptoms.

Morning Sickness

Your nausea may intensify when you're breastfeeding. In some cases, the physical process of letting down aggravates nausea, while in other cases, finding a position for the nursing child is the more likely trigger. Nausea, however, will not magically vanish just because you wean; it may simply be an inevitable symptom that plagues you regardless of your breastfeeding decision. Since it's important to eat well if you're breastfeeding this time around, see your doctor to discuss ways to combat severe nausea. In some cases, you may need to wean if you are not able to keep anything down. (For more information on morning sickness, consult my book *The Pregnancy Sourcebook*.)

Nipple Soreness

Remember when chapter 7 pointed out that some causes of nipple soreness are due to another pregnancy? Well, it's still true. Just as you experienced breast changes and nipple tenderness in your previous pregnancy, your next will be no exception. In fact, if nipple soreness persists and you've ruled out infections, weaning may be the only solution. (See chapter 7 for more information on nipple soreness.)

Moodiness

Apparently, it's very common to feel irritated, restless, and just plain antsy when you're breastfeeding during a pregnancy. No one really knows why this occurs, but it's important to be aware of these feelings. This may be nature's way of protecting the fetus or may be caused by a cross-circuiting of pregnancy and breastfeeding hormones. If these feelings interfere with breastfeeding, it may be time to wean until after the birth.

New Taste, New Product

Due to hormonal "staff changes" beyond your control, your milk will change in taste, quantity, and consistency. For example, during the last few months of pregnancy, the mature milk changes back into colostrum in preparation for the birth of another newborn. Some nursing toddlers don't mind the taste; others get really turned off. If your toddler doesn't mind the new flavor and consistency, there's no reason to stop breastfeeding. And no, your toddler will not exhaust your colostrum supply. You'll just make more.

As discussed earlier, all that estrogen coursing through your system will lower prolactin levels and hence your milk supply. That's why estrogen-containing contraceptives are discouraged. If your nursing baby is younger than a year and is breastfeeding exclusively, this decrease in milk production could affect that child's nutritional needs. Make sure you're keeping track of weight gain, wet diapers, and bowel movements. You may need to supplement your breast milk. (See chapter 6 for more details.)

The decrease in your milk may also cause your nursing child to self-wean. The process is gradual and natural, and the child will simply show more interest in other foods and liquids.

A common scenario to prepare for is one in which a nursing child who has self-weaned suddenly develops an appetite for breastfeeding once the new baby is born. At this point, you can decide whether you want to breastfeed the older child for comfort and supplementary nutrition. If you decide to breastfeed both children, or *tandem nurse*, read on.

TANDEM NURSING

Tandem nursing is often confused with breastfeeding during pregnancy, but it refers to breastfeeding two or more of your children when they're at *different* ages. In other words, breastfeeding twins is not tandem nursing. The most common configuration is to be breastfeeding a newborn and a toddler anywhere from one to two years of age. Deciding to tandem nurse is an incredibly individual decision that depends on a number of things:

- your physical health
- the age and health of your older, still-nursing child
- the health of your newborn
- your time
- your partner's feelings about the process
- your emotional comfort with the idea

When Is a Toddler Too Old?

The World Health Organization's guidelines recommend two years of breastfeeding (exclusive at least for the first six months, if possible, and at least four months). By these standards, no toddler is too old, and the decision to wean becomes an issue of individual preference and one that spills over into child-care psychology. Baby-led weaning (when the toddler gradually loses interest in breastfeeding) usually occurs naturally in the toddler stage anyway. If baby-led weaning doesn't occur as quickly as you'd like, you can lead the weaning. Some parents look upon weaning a toddler after the birth of a new baby as an opportunity for the toddler to learn about growing up and becoming more self-reliant (to the extent that a two- or three-year-old is self-reliant!).

Nursing Two under Two

The general rule is to nurse the youngest child first. You may also notice that the older child may suddenly want to nurse more often than before the baby was born. First, the milk is beginning to taste "better"—like the "breastmilk classic" brand the older child is used to. Second, your milk supply will have increased, making more milk available to the older child. Finally, the older child may be nursing for comfort and stability to cope with all the new life changes that the newborn sibling brings. You may find that the more insecure the older child feels, the more that child will want to nurse. This is normal and natural and may be an issue for a child psychologist to solve if it becomes a problem.

It's also important to remember that all those "getting started" issues discussed in earlier chapters, such as latch, positioning, and engorgement, may resurface depending upon how well the newborn is taking to the breast and how frequently your older child is nursing.

A common worry during tandem nursing is what to do when one of your children is ill. Usually, the older child's illness will trigger a protective instinct that may cause you to limit that child to one breast while you feed the newborn from the other. Or you may even feel like restricting breastfeeding or withholding breastfeeding from the older child. None of this is necessary. Because by the time your older child shows signs of a cold or flu, the newborn has already been exposed to the bug for several days. The colostrum will protect the newborn from catching more grown-up garden-variety ailments that either you or other family members might pass on.

Positions

Finding a comfortable position for your newborn will be similar to your search the last time around. Review chapter 4 for more information on positioning. If you're nursing two children simultaneously, review the section on positioning for nursing multiples for some pointers.

The only new information for you in terms of positioning is the fact that your older child will most likely be able to nurse in any position—no matter how awkward! In fact, the best plan is to make sure the newborn is comfortable and let the older child squirm his way to your breast. After a certain point, many older babies practically feed themselves.

Some women find that a baby sling or carrier not only makes tandem nursing easier but also makes raising the older child easier, allowing for hands-free feeding.

The Waiting Game

Older children who are still nursing will need to learn the concept of waiting: either waiting their turn or waiting for a more appropriate place to nurse if you're in public. This may be an easy thing to teach or may turn into an agonizing experience for the older child, causing you great stress.

How well your child responds to waiting depends on her age,

temperament, and frequency of breastfeeding. Some women find that the older child can handle waiting when nursing is restricted to certain places, while others do better when you restrict nursing to certain times. In contrast, some women report that asking the older child to wait even a few minutes is intolerable for that child. But often the same child will react in radically different ways depending on what time of day it is. The only solution is to experiment. And then experiment some more. Much of this waiting game has to do with life with a two-year-old. In fact, you may be familiar with this old joke: What's the difference between a two-year-old and a terrorist? You can *negotiate* with a terrorist!

I Changed My Mind

Tandem nursing may sound wonderful to you in theory, but once begun may turn into not such a wonderful practice after all. Many women reach the point at which they're "touched out." Too much cuddling, too much nursing, too much attention paid to the older child and the newborn can cause a real physical need to simply be left alone. Sometimes the solution is donating half an hour each day to solitude in the form of a bath, a walk, and so on. Sometimes the solution is to wean. The bottom line is that you must do what feels right to *you*. If tandem nursing is too overwhelming or unpleasant for you, it's time to wean.

chapter 11

WHAT YOU SHOULD KNOW ABOUT BABY MILK

hat would be your reaction if you were sent a case of free insulin for your healthy, *nondiabetic* newborn with the following pamphlet:

Babylin* artificial baby insulin is the next best thing to baby's own insulin. But baby's little pancreas sometimes cannot produce enough insulin for his little body. That's why we've developed Babylin. Doctors recommend Babylin is safe as an alternative or supplement for both diabetic babies and healthy babies. So if you're not sure baby's making enough insulin, you can be sure with Babylin. And when you fill out this coupon, we'll send you a free car seat. It's our way of saying we care.

Anyone who knows anything about the appropriate use of insulin and the dangers of giving insulin to a healthy person would be outraged at such an advertisement. If artificial insulin were injected into nondiabetic babies, they would go into insulin shock (severe hypoglycemia) and die. If you didn't know anything about human biology (and why would you unless you had formal training in medicine or nursing) and didn't know that a healthy pancreas makes insulin on supply and demand, you might be inclined to think that the Babylin product somehow improves on nature or is better for your child in some way. The pamphlet suggests that not by not giving supplemental or artificial insulin, a mother puts her baby's health at risk. If you were mother living in the Third World, you might also be influenced to think that if "Babylin" is given to First World babies, it must be better,

---

Babylin is a fictitious product. Any resemblance to a real product is purely coincidental.

healthier, or more scientific. What if you further discovered that the makers of Babylin were trying to buy support or endorsement from the medical establishment by regularly sponsoring medical conferences, offering research funding to scientists and medical researchers, and paying doctors substantial amounts of money for use of their names in ads and pamphlets?

The success of such an advertisement completely depends on the ignorance of its target market. The less educated the mother is about human biology, the easier it is to misinform her. The way to successfully market Babylin is to convince the public that there is a need for it. Babylin would certainly be required if a baby were not producing insulin. But the marketing campaign suggests that it's appropriate to give artificial insulin not just to babies who have a true medical need for it, but to those who do not.

The marketing campaign I've outlined for the fake product Babylin is modeled after a real baby product that is unnecessary most of the time. That product is baby formula, also known as artificial baby milk or breast milk substitutes.

HOW IT ALL BEGAN

Artificial baby milk was originally intended as a lifesaving product when there was no other way to nourish the baby. It was a product designed as a last resort but never intended for routine use. If you found Babylin an absurd product to be touting to mothers—experts who already understand human biology, human history, mammal behavior, and survival instincts—then the routine feeding of artificial baby milk to infants (99 percent of women are physically capable of breastfeeding) is just as absurd.

All health authorities urge women to breastfeed for at least one year and exclusively for at least six months, if possible. Despite this, $3 billion per year is spent in the United States on artificial baby milk; 38 percent of women in the United States never even attempt breastfeeding, while only 15 percent of women in the United States breastfeed their babies for a year. Artificial baby milk also costs at least $1,000 per year.

Worldwide, the marketing of artificial baby milk is responsible for roughly 4,000 infant deaths each day. These deaths occur because the marketing of the product (especially in areas where clean water or cow's milk is not affordable or available) entices the mother away from breastfeeding, exposing the baby to death from diarrhea or infections due to the absence of breastmilk.

The successful marketing of artificial baby milk is a socioeconomic story, not a medical or scientific one. In the social history of breastfeeding, aristocratic women would employ the services of a wet nurse. Wet nurses prior to the Industrial Revolution were usually married women whose husbands traveled. The wage was usually quite good for its day, and in cases of the very wealthy or royalty, the infants would be placed in the wet nurse's own home. Live-in wet nurses were also considered good jobs. In these cases, the wet nurse would be well fed and kept free from undue stress since it was understood at the time that stress interfered with milk letdown. Wet nursing was also a profession unwed mothers could turn to in an effort to support themselves and to help prevent another pregnancy.

Several factors led to a decline in wet nursing as a tradition and a profession. When the childbirth industry was taken over by male physicians during the nineteenth century, the belief that wet nurses spread syphilis and diseases to their charges began to take hold within society. This coincided with the theory that disease was spread by germs, which dominated scientific thought at the time. This led to a dramatic decline in the number of wet nurses and midwives, the very people who were knowledgeable about breastfeeding. In addition, the Industrial Revolution led to urbanization, immigration, and mass employment of women as factory workers. It also led to the industrialization of dairy farming, which resulted in large surpluses of whey, the waste product created in the manufacture of cow's milk. Artificial baby milk was first created from this one waste product, which could effectively be marketed to two distinct social groups: poor women who worked in factories (many of whom had once earned a better living wet nursing) and had no choice but to leave their babies at home; and rich women who were deprived of their wet nurses and considered themselves too delicate for breastfeeding. Thus, freedom from breastfeeding was seen as an attractive feature for both groups, and bottle-feeding emerged as a status symbol. Women who breastfed were considered "old fashioned" and not modern.

The term *formula* came into vogue around the turn of the nineteenth century. Various doctors began experimenting with different ingredients to try to make artificial milk closer to breastmilk. They would present their recipes as scientific formulas, and in the case of those who could afford it, babies would have an individual formula tailored to their digestive systems. In fact, in 1888, a prominent member of the American Medical Association noted that what nourishes one baby may kill the next baby. This business of tailored formulas went out of fashion quite soon because it was inconvenient, but the term was then adopted by various companies to make their product sound scientific. By the 1920s, the baby food industry was medicalized in partnership with commercial companies and doctors who invented their own special batches of artificial baby milk and benefited from royalties on sales.

As hospital births became the norm, hospital practices which discouraged breastfeeding became the norm, too. These practices included separating the mother and baby, routine bottle-feeding of artificial baby milk, or delaying introducing the baby to the breast when breastfeeding was desired by the mother. It was also routine practice to prescribe drugs that blocked the production of breast milk. Hospitals would be showered with free artificial baby milk, posters, toys, and gift baskets for mom from a myriad of manufacturers.

Not Created Equal

By the 1940s, the "equivalency position" was introduced into artificial baby milk marketing; artificial milk (evaporated, condensed, powdered, or specially formulated milk made from cow's or goat's milk) was sold as a substance that was "equal" in every way to breast milk, when it was not. By the late 1960s, the equivalency position evolved into the choice positioning, which coincided with the women's rights movement. Bottle-feeding was marketed as a woman's choice, designed to free her from her biology. While this appealed to the popular "biology is not destiny" argument made by many prominent feminist thinkers, unless a woman is truly informed about the dangers of not breastfeeding, she is not free to choose.

By the 1970s, study after study proved what breastfeeding advocates (who were considered radicals) were saying all along: breast is best. As advocacy groups began to grow, so did the "breast is best" message, and more women began to choose breastfeeding over bottle-feeding. As a result, the marketing of artificial baby milk became much more subtle. The companies produced booklets, pamphlets, and advertorials (an advertisement that looks like a regular editorial) about artificial baby milk and disguised it as "medical information" on breastfeeding, pregnancy, childbirth, and general childcare. Since these companies had more money to spend on advertising than the advocacy groups promoting breastfeeding, the literature about breastfeeding and bottle-feeding soon became controlled by the artificial baby milk companies.

Some of the common techniques used in the marketing literature includes slipping in doctors names to support distorted information about breast milk equivalency, vitamin supplementation, when to introduce solids, and charts and tables to give the literature a more scientific look. In company booklets and pamphlets, there is no mention of any particular brand, but the information on breastfeeding is inaccurate enough to discourage breastfeeding or make bottle-feeding attractive. Copy about breastfeeding is frequently accompanied by pictures of beautiful women bottle-feeding and beautiful babies being bottle-fed. Frequently, pictures of fathers bottle-feeding are used, suggesting that artificial baby milk promotes father-baby bonding. This literature is often provided to women as part of a "club pack" of other goodies: baby growth charts, posters, books, toys, games, audio tapes complete with a giant tin of free powdered artificial milk. "Pass-it-on" cards are frequently enclosed, encouraging new mothers to fill out a card so that her friends can also receive free gifts from the company.

Feeding the Nurses

The marketing of artificial baby milk also includes teaching hospital nursing staff how to discourage breastfeeding early, so that companies ensure that their product will sell. For example, maternity ward and neonatal nurses are frequently invited to events sponsored by the artificial baby milk companies. These events are then followed by a short presentation on product offerings, with lots of misinformation on scheduled feedings, lactation failure (which is highly unusual, and often caused by scheduled feedings), when to supplement a newborn, or when to discourage breastfeeding in certain women. Well-paid nutritionists, doctors, and other experts (often mothers themselves who use the company product on their own children) are frequent speakers at these events, too. Feeding newborns artificial milk or glucose water in hospitals is still routine and one of the surest ways to sabotage breastfeeding. Many studies have shown that a large percentage of women who want to breastfeed leave the hospital unable to do so as a result of hospital ward practices and staff ignorance.

Milk Marketing in the Third World

Like tobacco companies, artificial baby milk companies profit in the Third World. Because the product comes from the First World, it's assumed that it's more nutritious and safer for babies than breast milk. But given the fact that only one-third of the world has adequate sanitation and 99 percent of rural families and at least 50 percent of urban families in the Third World have no access to running water or uncontaminated water, artificial baby milk is often deadly to the child who is first, deprived of the immunity properties of breast milk, and second, exposed to deadly bacteria from contaminated water.

There is also the cost of the artificial milk product itself. In Nigeria, for example, the annual cost of artificial baby milk is equal to 264 percent of the minimum urban annual wage. Mothers go hungry in order to purchase this product. And this cost does not include the incidentals: clean water and fuel, or antibiotics and medical care if the baby suffers from diarrhea or infections. Of course, even if women in these regions can afford the artificial milk, they may lack the literacy skills to read the label and preparation instructions.

Even in the presence of HIV/AIDS, artificial baby milk is not a solution, but a dilemma. Unless a mother is HIV-positive, there appears to be no moral justification to sell artificial baby milk to the Third World. The situation is analogous to tobacco companies selling cigarettes to children and then denying that they are addictive.

POLICING ARTIFICIAL CLAIMS

Concerned over global infant mortality rates due to a decline in breastfeeding, the International Code of Marketing of Breastmilk Substitutes was created in 1981 to control inappropriate marketing practices. The code was drafted by WHO and UNICEF, representatives from governments, scientific experts, health workers, representatives from the infant food industry, representatives from consumer groups, and the International Baby Food Action Network (IBFAN), which remains the official "author." The final draft of the Code was approved by the World Health Assembly by 118 votes to 1. The United States was the only country to vote against the Code, fearing its repercussions on business.

What Does the Code Say?

The Code is designed to protect breastfeeding and control unethical or incorrect marketing practices. It's aimed at governments and companies and is intended as a minimum guideline for marketing practices. The products that come under the Code include artificial baby milk (or formula), other artificial milks (because these are sometimes used as baby milk), all baby foods and juices, feeding bottles, and nipples. By 1996, sixteen countries had simply adopted the Code into law, while twenty-six other countries had passed portions of the Code as law.

One of the most important yet most misinterpreted parts of this code deals with information and education, specifying that objective and consistent information must be provided to families about infant and child feeding. That means mixed messages such as "breastfeeding is best, but bottle-feeding is okay too" can be harmful. Artificial baby milk companies have then taken up the task of providing information on breastfeeding, stating that it is within their scope of duties. But it is not up to these companies to educate; this is the role of governments.

Under the Code, information and education materials must include complete information on the superiority of breast milk; proper nutrition for lactating women; how to prepare and maintain breastfeeding; the dangers of supplementation; how difficult it is to reverse the decision of not breast-feeding; and the proper instructions and use of artificial baby milk. Any information on artificial milk must include the social and financial implications of its use and health risks. No pictures or charts idealizing artificial milk can be included in the literature, either. The Code also stipulates:

- Information or educational materials, equipment, or product can only be donated with the written approval of the appropriate government authority or within government guidelines. (Company logos can appear, but no brand name can appear.) These donations can be distributed only through the health care system.

- No company material should be given directly to mothers.

- Health authorities should take appropriate measures to encourage and protect breastfeeding and promote the principles of this Code. (This means that hospitals must stop practices that discourage breastfeeding, such as giving supplemental feedings to infants unnecessarily, or separating mothers from their babies.)

- No facility of a health care system should be used for the purpose of promoting artificial baby milk.

- Facilities of health care systems should not be used for the display of products, such as posters, booklets, leaflets, brochures, feeding bottles, cot tags, stickers, clinic cards, prescription pads, and similar materials advertising artificial feeding.

- No company-supplied staff can be allowed to work in the health care system as "professional service representatives" or "mothercraft nurses." And, no company-supplied staff is to have contact with mothers.

- Demonstrating bottle-feeding with artificial baby milk can only be done by health workers or other community workers if necessary. These demonstrations are to target only those mothers or family members who medically require artificial baby milk. The demonstration must also include information on the risks of improper use.

- No free or low-cost supplies of artificial baby milk are to be distributed in any part of the health care system. Charitable donations of artificial baby milk, feeding bottles, or other such products may only be given by companies to orphanages and similar social welfare institutions but not to hospitals and maternity wards. And, they must be given only to babies in true medical need. Finally, the donations must last for as long as the baby needs them. (Note: Companies have been ignoring this provision and have been supplying almost unlimited quantities of free product to health care facilities. They have also been interpreting babies in need as babies whose mothers are going back to work.)

- Hospitals, clinics, and maternity wards must purchase their artificial baby milk as they would any other supply. (Note: Although the code stipulates no donations to such institutions, supplies are still being delivered through "back door" channels.)

- All information provided by companies to health professionals should be restricted to scientific and factual matters and should not suggest bottle-feeding is equivalent or superior to breastfeeding.

- No promotion to health workers is allowed, and no incentives (financial or material) are to be offered to health workers. Health workers must disclose whether they've received funding from any of these companies for fellowships, study tours, research grants, attendance at professional conferences, and so on. The companies must also disclose to whom they've granted funding. To prevent conflicts of interest, professionals working in child health cannot receive money, goods, or services from any of these companies.

- Health workers should not give samples of artificial baby milk to pregnant women, mothers of infants and young children, or members of their families.

Code Breaking

Just because this Code exists doesn't mean everyone abides by it. In fact, there are all sorts of ways around the Code to the dismay of its authors.

For example, companies are finding ways of marketing other kinds of infant foods that can interfere with breastfeeding but are not marketed as artificial baby milk. In Europe and parts of Asia and the Middle East, one company makes herbal teas for infants from as early as the first week of life. But since these teas contain over 90 percent sugar, they are not healthy for a baby and will interfere with breastfeeding. In Asia, Africa, and Latin America, other companies are pushing cereal and vegetable-based solid foods for the first month of life. But again, introducing solids too early will not only interfere with breastfeeding, but will cause the baby to lose vital energy and nutrients and may even expose him or her to contaminants. (For the record, solids are not necessary until the sixth month of life, and even then, should be introduced as a complement to ot a replacement for breast milk. Some artificial milk companies are even selling artificial milks just for mom, targeting pregnant and lactating women with special milks designed to give them special nutrients. New markets have also created opportunites for Code breaking. In Eastern Europe, for example, people are interested in anything Western so mothers are an easy market for artificial baby milk. Meanwhile, there is limited awareness about the Code by Eastern European health workers.

In Europe and the Third World, companies have begun to take the "dog food" approach, selling follow-up baby milk the way one would sell puppy food for the first six months and then regular dog food thereafter. Similarly, these follow-up milks are targeting babies four months and up; and the companies that make it deny that they're selling the same old artificial baby milk in a new tin. Once the consumer is hooked on the follow-up milk, it is recommended for infants up to twelve months, and some brands recommend these milks for up to three years. (In many cases, the system works more subtly: the child continues to "graduate" to different tins as he or she grows older.) Be it food or drink, for the record, the World Health Assembly, along with other health authorities, such as WHO and UNICEF, maintain that any food or drink given to the baby before it is nutritionally required interferes with breastfeeding, is not necessary, and is not to be promoted.

Bottle and nipple makers (pacifiers are categorized as nipples or teats) simply market their wares as if the Code did not apply to them. They continue to advertise directly to the public (which the Code forbids). They also give free samples and promotional gimmicks to parents. Most people assume that rubber nipples are safe products, but there have been reports of nitrosamines, a toxic family of compounds, found in rubber nipples and pacifiers. Nipples made of silicone are also being marketed, even though several babies have almost choked to death from broken pieces of silicone. Although pacifiers are very popular in the developed world, nonetheless, these are considered to be unnecessary and can put the baby at risk for diarrhea due to improper washing and hygiene.

THE LAST WORD

I hope that this book has at least helped you make an informed decision about breastfeeding and at best has given you the information and support you needed to *hang in there*. (See table 11-1.) When interviewing dozens of women across North America, I asked for words of advice. Overwhelmingly, the response was *Make sure you tell your readers that breastfeeding gets easier. Sure, it takes time at first, but so does formula-feeding.*

I'm particularly interested in getting your feedback about the quality and quantity of information in this book. Let me know what you NEED to know, so I can add more information to later editions. Write to me in care of the publisher. Breast milk is the best food you can give your baby. And in times of health-care reform and a threatened collapse of universal health care in countries that currently provide it, I strongly feel that breastfeeding is a matter of public health, private responsibility, and preventive health care.

Ideally, I hope you had this book with you during the last stages of pregnancy, since planning for breastfeeding is so important. But for those who picked up this book somewhere in the middle, I've carefully cross-referenced information so you don't miss anything. I've also provided a list of resources in the appendix where you can go for more information. This book is designed for breastfeeders of all ages and backgrounds. Read it, share the information with your friends, and take it with you to your doctor or baby's doctor. Good luck and good health.

Table 11-1

SOME ADVANTAGES FOR BREASTFEEDING

Best for baby

Reduces the incidence of allergies such as asthma and eczema

Economical—no waste

Antibodies—greater immunity to some infectious diseases

Stool inoffensive—hardly ever constipated

Temperature always ideal

Fresh milk—never goes off

Emotionally bonding

Ecologically sound

Digested easily—within two to three hours

Immediately available—no mixing required

Nutritionally optimal

Gastroenteritis greatly reduced

Source: International Baby Food Action Network, *Protecting Infant Health: A Health Workers' Guide to the International Code of Marketing of Breastmilk Substitutes, 8th edition.*

Table 11-2

SUMMARY OF THE INTERNATIONAL CODE OF MARKETING OF BREASTMILK SUBSTITUTES

1. No advertising of these products to the public.
2. No free samples to mothers.
3. No promotion of products in health care facilities, including no free or low-cost formula.
4. No company representatives to contact mothers.
5. No gifts or personal samples to health care workers. Health care workers should never pass products on to mothers.
6. No words or pictures idealizing artificial feeding, including pictures of infants, on the labels.
7. Information to health care workers must be scientific and factual.
8. All information on artificial infant feeding must explain the benefits and superiority of breastfeeding and the costs and hazards associated with artificial feeding.
9. Unsuitable products, such as sweetened condensed milk, should not be promoted for babies.
10. Manufacturers and distributors should comply with the Code's provisions even if countries have not acted to implement the Code.

Source: International Baby Food Action Network, *Protecting Infant Health: A Health Workers' Guide to the International Code of Marketing of Breastmilk Substitutes, 8th edition.*

WHERE TO GO FOR MORE INFORMATION

Note: Because of the volatile nature of many health and/or nonprofit organizations regarding funding and resources, some of these addresses and numbers may have changed since this list was compiled. I apologize for any inconvenience. If there are no known milk banks in your area, arrangements can be made on a "buddy system" through a local La Leche League if you wish to donate milk or require milk. In this case, the donor must undergo HIV and STD screening prior to donating milk.

Global Advocacy Groups

World Alliance for Breastfeeding
(WAVBA)
P.O. Box 1200, 10850
Penang, Malaysia
(604) 658-4816   Fax: (604) 657-2655

International Baby Food Action Network
(IBFAN) North America
129 Church Street
New Haven, Connecticut 06510

Distributing Donor Milk Banks for the United States and Canada

Mother's Milk Bank
c/o Professional Group
P.O. Box 5730
San Jose, CA 95150
(408) 998-4550

Triangle Mother's Milk Bank
Wake Medical Center
3000 New Bern Avenue
Raleigh, NC 27610
(919) 250-8599

Mother's Milk Bank
PSL Medical Center
1719 East 19th Avenue
Denver, CO 80218
(303) 869-1888

Community Human Milk Bank
Georgetown University Hospital
3800 Reservoir Road
Washington, DC 20007
(202) 784-6455

Wilmington Mother's Milk Bank
Christiana Hospital
P.O. Box 1665
Wilmington, DE 19579
(302) 733-2340

Regional Milk Bank
U Mass/Memorial
119 Belmont Street
Worcester, MA 01605
(508) 793-6005

Lactation Support Service
BC Children's Hospital
4480 Oak Street
Vancouver, BC, Canada V6H 3V4
(604) 875-2345 x7607

Products for Flat or Inverted Nipples

Maternal Concepts
P.O. Box 39
Spring Valley, WI 54767
(715) 778-4723   1-800-310-5817
www.snj.com\maternal
email: matcon@snj.com

For Information on Breast Implants

Food and Drug Administration
5600 Fishers Lane
Rockville, MD 20857
(301) 443-5006
1-800-532-4440

Life After Silicone
Hotline: (407) 622-5469

Public Citizen Health Research Group
2000 P Street NW
Washington, DC 20036
(202) 833-3000

Scleroderma Support Group
8852 Enloe Avenue
Garden Grove, CA 92644
(714) 892-5297

Occupational Health (Breastfeeding in the Workplace)

National Institute for Occupational
Safety and Health (NIOSH)
Mailstop R-11
4676 Columbia Parkway
Cincinnati, OH 45226
1-800-356-4674

(Also consult chapter 9.)

Occupational Safety and Health
Administration (OSHA)
Office of Information and Consumer
Affairs
Room N-3647
200 Constitution Avenue NW
Washington, DC 20210
(202) 219-8151

General Information

Note: Some of the following organizations accept money and funding from baby formula companies. Ask whether they accept money from baby formula companies before you accept advice, literature, and so on.

American College of Nurse-Midwives
818 Connecticut Avenue NW, Suite 900
Washington, DC 20006
(202) 728-9860

American Foundation for Maternal and Child Health
439 E. 51st Street, 4th floor
New York, NY 10022
(212) 759-5510

American Gynecological and Obstetrical Society
c/o James R. Scott, M.D.,
OB/GYN Dept., Rm. 2B200
University of Utah
50 North Medical Drive
Salt Lake City, UT 84132
(801) 581-5501

Federation for Children with Special Needs
31 Wilshire Park
Needham, MA 02192
(617) 482-2915

Food and Nutrition Information Center
National Agricultural Library, Rm. 304
Beltsville, MD 20705
(301) 344-3719

Food and Safety and Inspection Service
(202) 447-9351

Healthy Mothers, Healthy Babies Coalition
409 12th Street SW, Room 309
Washington, DC 20024-2188
(202) 863-2458

International Cesarean Awareness Network (ICAN)
276 Clarks
Summit, PA 18411
(717) 585-4226

International Childbirth Education Associates (ICEA)
Box 20048
Minneapolis, MN 55420
(612) 854-8660

International Lactation Consultant Association
201 Brown Avenue
Evanston, IL 60202
(708) 260-8874

La Leche League International and Breastfeeding Reference Library and Database
1400 North Meacham Road
Schaumburg, IL 60173-4840
(708) 519-7730   Fax: (708) 519-0035

Maternity Center Association
48 East 92nd Street
New York, NY 10128
(212) 369-7300

National Association of Childbearing Centers (NACC)
3123 Gottschall Road
Perkiomenville, PA 18074
(215) 234-8068

Public Information Center of the Enviornmental Protection Agency
(202) 382-2080

Useful Hotlines

American Academy of Allergy &
Immunology
1-800-822-ASMA or (414) 272-6071

American Diabetes Association
1-800-232-3472 or (703) 549-1500

American Lupus Society
1-800-331-1802 or (310) 542-8891

American Mental Health Fund
1-800-433-5959 or 1-800-826-2336

American Psychiatric Association
(202) 336-5700

ASK-A-NURSE (614) 293-5678

Association of Multi-Ethnic Americans
(510) 523-2632

Asthma & Allergy Foundation of
America 1-800-7-ASTHMA

Brewer Prenatal Nutrition Hotline
(802) 388-0276

Calcium Information Line
1-800-321-2681 (Established in 1991 by
The Calcium Information Center, a
component of the Clinical Nutrition
Research Units of the New York
Hospital; Cornell Medical Center and
Memorial Sloan-Kettering Cancer
Center; and Oregon Health Sciences
University.)

General Information
1-800-4-A-BIRTH

Healthy Mothers, Healthy Babies
(202) 638-5577

Journal of American Medical
Association Calcium Report
1-800-753-0352 x707, or contact Anne
FitzSimons (212) 326-9800

Juvenile Diabetes Association
1-800-223-1138 or (212) 889-7575

Lupus Foundation of America
1-800-558-0121 or (301) 670-9292

Lyme Aid 1-800-886-LYME (Lyme
disease)

Mothers of Asthmatics (703) 385-4403

National Aids Information
Clearinghouse 1-800-458-5231

National Aids Network (202) 293-2437

National Association for Sickle Cell
Anemia
1-800-421-8453 or (203) 736-5455

National Council on Alcoholism and
Drug Dependence
1-800-423-4673 or (212) 206-6770

National Down Syndrome Society
1-800-221-4602 or (212) 460-9330

National Heart, Blood & Lung Institute
(310) 496-4236

National Herpes Hotline
(919) 361-8488

National HIV and Aids Information
Service 1-800-342-AIDS

National Immunizations Campaign
(202) 338-7227

National Maternal & Child Health
Clearinghouse (703) 821-8955

Pregnancy Riskline 1-800-822-2229

Sudden Infant Death Syndrome Alliance
1-800-221-7437

General Information for Canada

B.C. Breastfeeding Centre
690 West 11th Avenue
Vancouver, B.C. V5Z 1M1
(604) 875-4678   Fax: (604) 875-5017

La Leche League Canada
P.O. Box 29, 18C Industrial Drive
Chesterville, Ontario K0C 1H0
1-800-665-4324   (613) 448-1842
Fax: (613) 448-1845

The Hospital for Sick Children
Breastfeeding Clinic
555 University Avenue
(416) 813-5757
(A list of other Ontario Breastfeeding
Clinics is provided when you call this
number.)

INFACT Canada
6 Trinity Square
Toronto, Ontario M5G 1B1
(416) 595-9819   Fax: (416) 591-9355

Vancouver Women's Health Collective
175 West 85th Avenue, Suite 219
Vancouver, B.C. V5L 2Y7
(604) 736-5262

Women's College Hospital
Breastfeeding Clinic
76 Grenville Street
Toronto, Ontario M5S 1B2
(416) 323-6526
(A list of other Ontario Breastfeeding
Clinics is provided when you call this
number.)

Breastfeeding Online

Through the Internet, you can participate in newsgroups and bulletin boards (public forums) on prenatal or postpartum health. These can be accessed through either independent internet providers, or through an interactive computer service, such as CompuServe, Prodigy, or America Online (AOL).

Literature searches are great ways of getting specific information. Medline is the best for search service for medical journal articles (many of which are extremely technical). Compuserve, Prodigy, or AOL all give you access to Medline. Medline is also available through many public and university libraries throughout North America.

Another way of accessing good information is through a web browser, such as Netscape. By web browsing, you can go to various sites in cyberspace to find your information. When you don't know the worldwide web (www) address, you can use a search engine, such as Yahoo or Webcrawler, to search for what you want by simply typing in your topic. The more specific you can be in your search, the better. For example, if you want information on breast pumps, don't type "breastfeeding" but "breast pumps." A search engine is essentially an "index" to the Internet.

Once the search engine completes its search, a list of various sites will come up onscreen. These sites will range from promotional web sites from health food stores to university bulletin boards, to pepperings of articles. When you go to a site, you can save or print the information. Flashing text (called hypertext) is a sign that you'll get more information when you click on it. This may even link you to other sites on the Internet. A good resource to get is Internet for Dummies, which will walk you through Internet access step-by-step. Here are a couple of sites to get you started:

www.storksite.com

http://nlights.net/jclark/bfeed.htm
(An excellent "starting point" home page for breastfeeding information with dozens of links to other excellent homepages.)

Glossary

Note: This list is not exhaustive. These are not literal dictionary definitions but rather definitions created solely for the context of this book. Any resemblance to definitions found in other glossaries or dictionaries is purely coincidental.

Adenitis: An inflammation of the ducts within the breast. The infection starts in the milk spaces due to poor emptying of part of the breast, resulting in "milk stasis," in which the milk hangs around longer than it should.

Alveoli: Grapelike clusters of glandular tissue that help to synthesize milk out of blood.

Arching baby: A common and frustrating problem where the baby arches his or her head and body away from the breast and screams every time he or she begins to nurse.

Areola: The darkened part of the breast out of which the nipple protrudes. The areola darkens during pregnancy, later serving as a "bull's eye target" to better allow for the newborn to find the center of the breast. The pattern of pressure and release of the baby's mouth on the areola stimulates nerve pathways from the nipple to the brain to release the hormone prolactin into the bloodstream.

The Baby-Friendly Hospital Initiative: A worldwide effort, led by UNICEF and WHO (World Health Organization), to make hospitals "baby-friendly," wherein they adopt practices that support breastfeeding.

Baby-led weaning: When the baby loses interest in breastfeeding on his or her own.

Bilirubin: The yellow pigment that results as the baby breaks down old red blood cells to make way for new ones.

Bleb: A whitish, tender area under the areola, which looks like milk under the skin. This milk has somehow become trapped, causing the nipple and areola to become inflamed.

Breast herpes: Herpes simplex virus (HSV) I or II associated with sores above the waist. Mothers exposed to HSV can develop herpes sores on the nipples.

Breast milk jaundice (BMJ): This rarer form of jaundice, clinically termed late-onset jaundice, is thought to be triggered by something in the breast milk itself.

Breast shells: Also called milk cups, breast cups, breast shields, or Woolwich shields, breast shells are made of hard, lightweight plastic resembling an areola with a hole in the center for either a flat or inverted nipple to stick out of. Designed to be worn prior to delivery or between feedings to "train" an inverted or flat nipple to come out. Not recommended!

Candida albicans and monilia: The two organisms responsible for yeast infections in the mouth or nipple.

Cellulitis: An inflammation of the cellular breast tissue occurring when the lobular connective tissue is infected.

Chronic subareolar abscess: An uncommon bacterial infection of the sebaceous glands around the nipples.

Colostrum: Produced during the first few days of breastfeeding, colostrum contains complex immunological proteins, living white blood cells, and factors that activate bowel function. It nourishes the baby until the mature breast milk comes in.

Combination oral contraceptive: An oral contraceptive containing both estrogen and progesterone.

Conjunctivitis: Pinkeye.

Contraindicated: Unsafe, rather than "not indicated."

Cyclical breast pain: Premenstrual breast and nipple tenderness.

Cystine and taurine: Two important amino acids found in breast milk that are essential to the baby's brain development.

Donor milk: Breast milk donated by a third party.

Ductules: Branchlike tubes extending from the alveoli. Each of these ductules empties into larger ducts called mammary ducts.

Engorgement: Being overfilled or stuffed with milk.

Exocrine glands: Glands that produce a product used outside of the bloodstream. Breasts are exocrine glands in which the product is not used by the body but continues the work of the placenta which nourishes a fetus.

Flat nipples: A condition in which the nipple does not become erect when stimulated or cold.

Follicle stimulating hormone (FSH): Stimulates the ovary to produce estrogen and then progesterone at ovulation, triggering puberty.

Formula: Artificially manufactured breast milk, also called artificial baby milk.

Galactocele: A lacteal or milk cyst.

Galactosemia: A serious condition in which the liver enzyme that normally converts galactose to glucose (a simple sugar) is missing. Without it, the baby is unable to metabolize lactose and can suffer from severe symptoms that include vomiting, weight loss, cataracts, and even mental impairment.

Hand-expression funnel: A device used to express breast milk that is made of hard, lightweight plastic and doesn't require batteries or electricity.

Hypoglycemia: Low blood sugar.

Hypolactation: Poor milk production.

Hypothyroidism: An underactive thyroid gland.

Impetigo: A bacterial infection that can cause symptoms of burning and irritation.

Infant lactose overload: Occurs when the mother makes more milk than the baby needs or can handle.

Inverted nipples: A condition in which the nipples retract into the breast rather than protrude when the areola is compressed.

Jaundice: A baby who turns yellow has jaundice. With normal jaundice (physiological jaundice), the skin turns yellow because the red blood cells that are being retired from service result in the production of a yellow pigment called bilirubin. Neonatal jaundice is an extremely common problem, affecting roughly 50 percent of all normal, full-term infants within the first week of life. Breastfeeding is usually the best medicine.

Kegel exercises: Developed to improve the grip of the vagina, Kegels involve a repeated contraction of the muscle that starts and stops the urinary stream.

Lactagogues: Medications that trigger the breasts to make (more) milk.

Lactational amenorrhea (LAM): A natural cessation of the menstrual cycle during exclusive breastfeeding. Lactational amenorrhea generally lasts at least six months. It is considered to be an effective form of birth control if the baby is less than six months old, if the mother has not experienced any vaginal bleeding after the fifty-sixth postpartum day, and if she is exclusively (or almost exclusively) breastfeeding.

Lactational mastitis: Infection of the milk-producing breast.

Lactation consultant (LC): The equivalent of a breastfeeding midwife, an LC is trained to help new mothers learn the technique of breastfeeding, provide information about breastfeeding, and solve problems that arise during breastfeeding.

Lactiferous sinuses: Located underneath the nipple and areola, this is where the milk collects and waits for the baby to start suckling.

Lactose intolerance: A condition caused by an absence of the enzyme lactase, which breaks down lactose into simple sugars, necessary for digestion. Babies are born with lactase in their intestinal systems, and only in very rare cases do they lack the enzyme.

Latching on: A term used to describe a baby who is properly positioned and suckling at the breast. A good latch entails the baby taking the areola into his or her mouth along with the nipple. A poor latch makes feeding difficult and is the most common reason for sore nipples and pain during nursing.

Leaking: When milk leaks from the breast; often caused when a mother sees, hears, or even thinks of her baby.

Lipase: Present in human milk, the enzyme lipase is also found in the breastfed baby's intestine. Lipase breaks down the fat from triglycerides (the basic ingredient of all fat) into fatty acids and glycerol.

Lobe: Comprised of "stems" or mammary ducts, there are fifteen to twenty-five lobes in the breast, and each lobe consists of twenty to forty lobules (a smaller milk duct with its supporting alveoli).

Mammary ducts: Also called lactiferous ducts, these stems connect the ductules to the nipple.

Mammary glands: Breasts—these glands that define a woman's biological class. The word mammal comes from the term mammary gland.

Manual pumps: Used to express breast milk, the best of these are cylinder-type pumps, where one cylinder fits inside another, with a rubber gasket acting as a seal between. Suction and pressure are created when the inner cylinder is pulled out, drawing the milk into the outer cylinder or a separate collection bottle.

Mastalgia: Breast pain.

Meconium: The waste of a fetus found in the womb.

Milk letdown: Also called the "letdown reflex" or the "milk-ejection reflex," milk letdown occurs when the myoepithelial cells actively squeeze the milk out of the breast into the milk sinuses.

Milk ridge: A line made up of human breast tissue, which runs from the armpit all the way down to the groin, and which begins to develop in the sixth week of fetal life.

Montgomery glands: Located in the areola, these glands act as tiny muscles that contract and widen to help get the milk out.

Mother-led weaning: Also called "premature weaning," this process begins when the mother decides to wean before the baby does.

Nasogastric tube: Used to feed larger premies, this device is similar to the nasojejunal tube, only it sends the milk directly to the baby's stomach.

Nasojejunal tube: A nasal tube designed to provide constant, intravenous nourishment.

Newborn hypoglycemia: A result of the baby's blood sugar being too low. This situation can occur if a mother had either a difficult pregnancy, involving perhaps toxemia or gestational diabetes, or a long, difficult delivery.

Nipple: The point at which all mammary ducts meet, the nipple is made up of delicate nerve endings which narrow at the nipple opening or pore.

Nipple confusion: A term used to describe a baby who "forgets" how to suckle from a real nipple as a result of sucking on a fake one.

Nipple shields: Soft latex, silicone, or rubber nipples designed to be worn over the nipples during feedings. Shields, which destroy a mother's milk supply, were invented to help women with sore nipples continue nursing.

Noncyclical breast pain: Usually anatomical rather than hormonal, with cysts being the probable cause of discomfort. This type of pain should be checked out by a doctor.

Nonlactational mastitis: A bacterial breast infection found in nonlactating women.

Nursing strike: When a baby suddenly refuses to breastfeed; seems perfectly healthy otherwise; and will feed via cup, spoon, or bottle.

Overactive letdown: Sometimes called "forceful milk ejection reflex," an overactive letdown can be just as problematic as a poor letdown or a deficient milk supply.

Oxytocin: Released by nipple stimulation, oxytocin is the hormone that not only triggers milk letdown, but also uterine contractions, which researchers say enhance sexual sensation.

Pathologic jaundice: This rare form of jaundice occurs when something causes the baby's red blood cells to break down faster than normal, causing bilirubin levels to rise faster and higher than normal.

Phenylketonuria (PKU): An inherited metabolic disorder that leads to mental impairment if left untreated. Here, the baby is unable to metabolize the amino acid phenylalanine, present in breast milk, which prevents normal brain and central nervous system development.

Phototherapy: A treatment used to treat severe jaundice, phototherapy involves placing the baby in direct sunlight or under a special fluorescent light in the blue-to-white range known as a "bililight." The light actually helps to break down the bilirubin through the skin.

Plugged ducts: Also known as the "plug," this term usually refers to ducts plugged at the nipple level, but a plug can also occur higher up in the breast, often the result of scarring or constriction rather than thickened milk, which causes the plug around the nipple.

Prolactin: Also called the "mothering hormone," prolactin is released by the pituitary gland and is crucial for breastfeeding.

Prostaglandins: Another ingredient in breast milk. During menstruation, prostaglandins, a chemical secreted by our tissues, pushes out the uterine lining each month. Prostaglandins also help the baby's digestive tract move more smoothly.

Pyloric stenosis: A serious condition that indicates a structural problem with the tube that connects the stomach to the intestine. Symptoms usually develop between two to eight weeks of age and are usually more common in firstborn white male babies.

Raynaud's syndrome: Raynaud's syndrome can develop where there is nipple damage of some kind. The nipple turns white and is extremely sensitive during and after feedings.

Relactation: A process undertaken by the mother who decides to resume breastfeeding (with either the same or another child) after she has weaned one child already.

Secretory glands: Glands, like the breasts, that secrete fluids.

SIDS: Sudden infant death syndrome.

Subclinical mastitis: Mild mastitis.

T-E fistula: Fistula refers to an abnormal tunnel that links two internal organs. A T-E fistula stands for tracheo (windpipe)-esophogeal (food pipe) fistula, an abnormal linking of the windpipe and the esophagus.

Thrush: A yeast infection that can cause symptoms of burning and irritation.

Tongue-tied: A baby who is tongue-tied has a short frenulum, and the tongue will rise up in a heart shape instead of a smooth curve when he or she cries. This is easily fixed by having a pediatrician clip the fold of tissue under the baby's tongue.

Weak suck: A baby with a weak suck doesn't have a structural problem at work but is having difficulty developing his or her suckling skill.

Wet nurse: Popular between the seventeenth and mid-nineteenth centuries, wet nurses were engaged by mothers considered too frail to produce "good milk." Wet nurses stayed "wet" by continually breastfeeding after they themselves had children.

Witch's milk: A term used to describe a newborn's ability to produce milk. This condition generally disappears in a couple of weeks, as the baby is weaned from the mother's hormones.

$\mathcal{B}$IBLIOGRAPHY

Altman, Lawrence K. "A Protest, AIDS Experts Quit Journal of Medicine." *The New York Times* (November 15, 1997).

Armstrong, H. "Feeding Low Birthweight Babies: Advances in Kenya." *Journal of Human Lactation* 3 (1987):34–37.

Arsenault, M.D., C.C.F.P, I.B.C.L.C., Gillian. Interview, 1995.

———. Breastfeeding: The Physician's Vade Mecum. 1994, unpublished as of this writing.

———. "You Learn the Darndest Things When You Have Kids, or What I Have Learned about Breastfeeding." *BC Health and Disease Surveillance* 2, no. 10 (September 13, 1993).

"Bedsharing, Breastfeeding Affect SIDS Risk." *Reuters* (August 4, 1997).

"Breastfeeding Affects PCB Cancer Risk." *Reuters* (August 21, 1997).

"Breastfeeding Recommended as Best." *Pediatrics* 100(6): 1035–39 (1997).

"Breastfeeding in the Workplace: Safety Considerations." *BC Health and Disease Surveillance* 3, no. 2 (February 7, 1994).

Bruning, Nancy. *Breast Implants: Everything You Need to Know.* Alameda, Calif.: Hunter House, 1992.

Crawford, M. "The role of essential fatty acids in neural development: implications for perinatal nutrition." *American Journal of Clinical Nutrition* 57: 703S-710S.

Carty, R.N., M.S.N., C.N.M., Elaine McEwan. "Resuming Intimacy: Couples Need to Express Their Love." *Best Wishes* 44, no. 3 (Fall, Winter 1992).

Dunley, Ruth. "Smoking ruins breast milk: equivalent of 20 cigarettes can be passed on to infants." *The Ottawa Citizen* (August 2, 1997).

Fayerman, Pamela. "Employees win right to breastfeed at work." *The Vancouver Sun* (August 12, 1997).

Ferguson, Anne E., et al. "Breastfeeding Infants Who Were Extremely Low Birth Weight." *Pediatrics* 100(6) (December 1997).

Fergusson, David M., and L. John Horwood. "Breastfeeding and Later Cognitive and Academic Outcomes." *Pediatrics* 101(1) (January 1998).

Flick, Jonathan, A. "Silicone Implants and Esophageal Dysmotility: Are Breast-fed Infants at Risk?" *JAMA* 271, no. 3 (January 19, 1994).

Freed, M.D., M.P.H., Gary L. "Breastfeeding: Time to Teach What We Preach." *JAMA* 269, no. 2 (January 13, 1993).

Frinton, M.D., Vera. "Your Changing Body: The Postpartum Period." *Best Wishes*, 44, no. 3 (Fall, Winter 1992).

Good, Judy. "Breastfeeding the Baby with Down Syndrome." La Leche League International, Inc. Publication No. 23, 1987.

—————. "The Diabetic Mother and Breastfeeding." La Leche League International, Inc. Information Sheet No. 17, 1987.

Grady, Edith, "Nursing My Baby with a Cleft of the Soft Palate." La Leche League International, Inc., Publication No. 22, 1989.

Hardman, R.N., Nancy L., and Lynn Jones, R.N., M.H.Sc., "The First Three Weeks: 20 Questions about Those First 20 Days." *Best Wishes* 45, no. 3 (Fall, Winter 1993).

Huml, Susan C., I.B.C.L.C. "Cracked Nipples in the breastfeeding mother: looking at an old problem in a new way." *Advance for Nurse Practitioners* (April 1995).

"Innocenti Declaration on the Protection, Promotion and Support of Breast-feeding." Document published by WHO/UNICEF at the policy-makers' meeting on "Breastfeeding in the 1990s: A Global Initiative" held at the Spedale degli Innocenti, Florence, Italy, July 30–August 1, 1990.

International Baby Food Action Network. *Protecting Infant Health: A Health Workers' Guide to the International Code of Marketing of Breastmilk Substitutes, 8th ed.* (November 1996).

Johanson, R.N., Sue. Interview with sex consultant, 1994.

Kennedy, K.I., R. Rivera, and A.S. McNeilly. "Consensus Statement on the Use of Breastfeeding as a family planning method." *Contraception* 39(5): 477–96 (1989).

Kesaree, Nirmala, MRCP, FRCP, C.R. et al., "Treatment of Inverted Nipples Using a Disposable Syringe." *Journal of Human Lactation* 9, no. 1 (1993).

Kramer, Matthew F., et al. "Breastfeeding Reduces Maternal Lower Body Fat." *Journal of the American Dietetic Association* 93 (April 1993).

La Leche League Canada. "Breastfeeding and Sexuality." Reprint no. 82, 1985.

———. "Can Breastfeeding Become the Cultural Norm?" Publication No. 61, 1989.

———. "Establishing Your Milk Supply." Reprint No. 81, 1989.

———. "Increasing Your Milk." Publication No. 85, 1988.

———. "Medications for the Nursing Mother." Publication No. 21, 1991.

———. "Sore Breasts." Publication No. 29, 1993.

La Leche League International, Inc. "Breastfeeding after a Cesarean Birth." Publication No. 80, 1988.

———. "Breastfeeding and Fertility." Publication No. 87, 1991.

———. "Breastfeeding Twins." Publication No. 52, 1991.

———. "Does Breastfeeding Take Too Much Time?" Publication No. 63, 1989.

———. "Newborn Jaundice." Publication No. 25, 1989.

———. "Nipple Confusion—Overcoming and Avoiding This Problem." Publication No. 32, 1992.

———. "Nursing with Breast Implants." Publication No. 24, 1992.

———. "Nutrition and Breastfeeding." Publication No. 159, 1994.

———. "Persistent Diarrhea: Could It Be Lactose Intolerance?" Publication No. 31, 1992.

———. "Positioning Your Baby at the Breast." Publication No. 107, 1987.

———. "Practical Hints for Working and Breastfeeding." Publication No. 83, 1991.

———. "Sore Nipples." Publication No. 28, 1989.

———. "When Babies Cry." Publication No. 20, 1991.

———. "When You Breastfeed Your Baby the First Week." Publication No. 124, 1993.

———. *The Womanly Art of Breastfeeding.* 4th ed. Franklin Park, Ill.: La Leche League International, 1987.

———. *The Womanly Art Of Breastfeeding.* 35th ed. Franklin Park, Ill.: La Leche League International, 1991.

Lander, M.D., F.R.C.P. (C), Debra. Interview, 1993.

Lazar, M.D., F.R.C.P. (C), F.A.C.P, Matthew. Interview with pediatrician/neonatal specialist, 1994.

"Letters to the Editor." *JAMA* 272, no. 10 (September 14, 1994): 767–770.

Levine, M.D., Jeremiah, J., and Norman T. Ilowite, M.D. "Sclerodermalike Esophageal Disease in Children Breast-fed by Mothers with Silicone Breast Implants." *JAMA* 271, no. 3 (January 19, 1994).

Love, M.D., Susan, and Karen Lindsey. *Dr. Susan Love's Breast Book*. New York: Addison-Wesley Publishing, 1991.

McKenna, James J., et al. "Bedsharing Promotes Breastfeeding." *Pediatrics* 100(2): 214–19 (August 1997).

Mardya, L., et al. "Breast-Feeding Lowers the Frequency and Duration of Acute Respiratory Infection and Diarrhea in Infants under Six Months of Age." *The Journal of Nutrition* 127(3):436–43 (March 1997).

Meintz Maher, I.B.C.L.C., Susan. *An Overview of Solutions to Breastfeeding and Sucking Problems*. La Leche League International, Inc., Publication No. 67, 1988.

Mohrbacher, I.B.C.L.C., Nancy, and Julie Stock, B.A., I.B.C.L.C. *The Breastfeeding Answerbook*. Franklin Park, Ill.: La Leche League International, 1991.

Morales, Karla, and Charles B. Inlander. *Take This Book to the Obstetrician with You*. New York: Addison-Wesley Publishing, 1991.

Mortimer, Jasper. "Tomb of Tutankhamen's wet nurse discovered near Cairo." *Associated Press* (December 7, 1997).

Newman, Jack. "Breastfeeding Problems Associated with Early Introduction of Bottles and Pacifiers." *Journal of Human Lactation* 6, no. 2 (1990): 59–63.

———. "How to know whether a health provider is breastfeeding or not," handout #18 (November 1996).

Nilsson, Ingeborg. "Sweden's Baby-Friendly Initiative." *UNICEF Quarterly* 992, no. 4 (October/December 1992).

Noble, Elizabeth, and Leo Sorger, M.D., F.A.C.O.G. *Having Twins*. Boston: Houghton Mifflin Company, 1991.

Palmer, Gabrielle. *The Politics of Breastfeeding*. London: Pandora Press, 1993.

Perez, A., M.H. Labbok, and J.T. Queenan. "Clinical Study of the Lactational Amenorrhoea Method for Family Planning." *The Lancet* 339(8799): 968–70 (1992).

Peters, R.N., Dawn. "Grandmother-to-Grandmother: A Word about Breast-feeding." *Best Wishes* 44, no. 3 (Fall, Winter 1992).

"Price Waterhouse Introduces Special Program for New Mothers." *PRNewswire*, Dec. 9, 1997.

Renfrew, Mary, Chloe Fisher, and Suzanne Arms. *Bestfeeding: Getting Breastfeeding Right for You.* Berkeley, Calif.: Celestial Arts, 1990.

Riordan, Jan. *A Practical Guide to Breastfeeding.* Boston: Jones and Bartlett Publishers, 1991.

Rooney, Kate. "Breastfeeding the Chronically Ill Child." La Leche League Canada, Publication No. 51, 1991.

Rosenthal, M. Sara. *The Fertility Sourcebook.* Los Angeles: Lowell House, 1995.

———. *The Gynecological Sourcebook.* Los Angeles: Lowell House, 1994.

———. *The Pregnancy Sourcebook.* Los Angeles: Lowell House, 1994.

Sears, M.D., William. *The Fussy Baby.* New York: Penguin Books, 1989.

"Secondhand Smoke Puts Children at Risk." *Reuters* (February 10, 1998).

"Silicone Breast Implants and Breast-Feeding: Commentaries." *Pediatrics,* (July 22, 1994).

Staseson, R.N., B.Sc.N., Sharon. "Post Partum Blues: What to Expect." *Best Wishes* 45, no. 3 (Fall, Winter 1993).

Stevenson-Smith, Fay, "After the Birth, (Recovering from Childbirth)." *Parents' Magazine* 68 (March 1993).

Stolberg, Sheryl Gay, "U.S. Ends Overseas H.I.V. Studies Involving Placebos." *The New York Times* (February 19, 1998).

Swanson, Leila. "Talking about Twins." *Best Wishes* 45, no.3 (Fall, Winter 1993).

"Take the Baby-Friendly Initiative!" UNICEF House booklet, 1994.

"10 Great Reasons to Breastfeed." Ministry of National Health and Welfare, Ministry of Supply and Services, pamphlet, Canada, 1990.

"10 Valuable Tips for Successful Breastfeeding." Ministry of National Health and Welfare, Ministry of Supply and Services, pamphlet, Canada, 1991.

UNAIDS. "Prevention of HIV Transmission from Mother-to-Child: Meeting on Planning for Programme Implementation." Statement made in Geneva, Switzerland (March 23–24, 1998).

UNAIDS press release. Joint Statement by The Centers for Disease Control and Prevention (CDC), The Joint United Nations Programme on HIV/AIDS

(UNAIDS), The National Institutes of Health (NIH), and The Agence Nationale de Recherche sur le SIDA (ANRS). Atlanta (February 18, 1998).

UNAIDS 1997 World AIDS Campaign. Posted to the Internet as www.us.un-aids.org (November 3, 1997).

"UNICEF Board Sets June 1994 Deadline." BFHI News, June, 1992.

Williams, A.F., Department of Child Health, St. Georges Hospital, London, UK, "Silicone Breast Implants, Breastfeeding, and Scleroderma." *The Lancet* 343 (April 23, 1994).

Wisner, K.L., et al. "Antidepressant treatment during breast-feeding." *American Journal of Psychiatry* 153(9): 1132–7 (1996).

INDEX